The Computer Diet

Metric Edition

Vincent W. Antonetti, PhD

NoPaperPress, LLC

Contents

Index of Tables

1. Introduction

The original hard-cover book *The Computer Diet*, published in 1973, was very well received and critically acclaimed. But now portions of the book are out of date. So at the insistence of some researchers and nutritionists who still refer to the original book and the editors at NoPaperPress, I agreed to write an updated version, and published it as an eBook in a first-time metric edition.

My interest in fitness, nutrition and eventually weight control started when I was twelve years old. My uncle, who was exactly ten years older than I was, had just been discharged from the U.S. Army. He decided to join a gym and I begged him to take me along. There were no fancy health clubs in those days – at least none that I knew of. The "gym" in reality was a converted three-car garage equipped with a heater. But inside there were some serious weight lifters. The members were not thrilled to have a twelve-year old kid in their midst. But the owner of the "gym" was an army buddy of my uncle, so he allowed me to join. He gave me a basic workout routine; stationed me in a corner and told me not to speak unless spoken to.

In that corner I did curls, presses, dead lifts, squats, shrugs, rows and got stronger. I also listened to the guys talk about what they ate and why they trained as they did. In due course I started to ask questions and got hooked on fitness and nutrition. I read every nutrition and exercise book in our local library. But after six months my family moved from an apartment to a one-family house with a detached-garage in the back, which I converted into a "gym" for myself and my new neighborhood friends.

How It All Started
Fast forward about twenty years. "We guarantee a weight loss of one kilo per week," read a newspaper advertisement sponsored by a weight control company. My wife wanted to lose five kilos and decided to attend a meeting.

Later, as my wife and I discussed what had transpired at the meeting, she said, "There was one point that didn't make sense. When I asked how long I would continue to lose one kilo a week," the speaker answered, 'for as long as you stay on the diet.' "My wife laughed when I remarked, "That would mean one year on that diet and you would disappear!"

We both concluded that what must happen in time is that weight loss must taper off. I then asked if the same diet was suggested for everyone. "Yes," she replied, "and everyone is supposed to lose two pounds per week." I continued, "That really doesn't make sense. In effect what they are saying is: if you and, for example, a professional American football player went on the same diet, both of you would lose weight at the same rate."

Intuitively, it seemed to me that if my wife and a 120 kilo football player were on the same diet, the football player would practically be starving and would certainly lose more weight than would my wife.

At that time, I had stopped smoking and had promptly gained five kilos. I was still gaining when I joined a YMCA. The exercise made me feel healthy and fit but I didn't lose weight.

As I recall, it was the conversation with my wife and my inability to lose weight that first aroused my interest in weight control. During the next five years, this casual interest grew into an after-hours research project, a literature search, a mathematical analysis, publication of a scientific paper, and in 1973 *The Computer Diet*.

Research

I began in the late 1960s by reading every diet book on the market. Frankly, I was not satisfied. The books were contradictory and because I am an engineer, I found they lacked the sort of quantitative information I was searching for. As a result, I gravitated toward the scientific literature. What I hoped to discover was a weight-loss predictive formula, or equation. I read books on physiology, nutrition, and then the latest research papers. And I found no such equation. I also began to correspond with scientists at leading universities.

My literature search revealed a tremendous amount of on-going weight control research but again no weight-loss predictive equation. There seemed to be two fundamentally different schools of thought concerning the nature of weight loss. One view argued that "calories do count," or in more scientific terms, that weight loss was governed by a fundamental concept of physics called the conservation of energy, discussed in greater detail in **Chapter 2** page 15. The contrary view, in brief, was that certain foods or food combinations had special qualities that cause weight to be lost more rapidly than would be predicted by the conservation of energy principle. I appraised both sides and the more deeply I read, the more convinced I became that the "calories-do-count" faction had it right. It seemed perfectly reasonable to me that the human metabolism should obey the conservation of energy – as does everything else in nature!

I further reasoned that if the conservation of energy applies to humans, it should be possible do a mathematical analysis of weight change in human beings. For years researchers have recognized that weight change depends on, at the very least, age, gender, height, weight, amount of physical activity, caloric intake and time. Unfortunately, the relationship of these factors to weight change had never been mathematically established. With the background in physiology and nutrition I had gained over the years through my reading, plus my engineering-mathematics training and experience, I set myself the task of developing the equations involved in weight change.

That I would attempt such an analysis is not as unusual as it might appear. There are a relatively large group of engineers working in a field that falls somewhere between medicine and engineering called bio-medical engineering. For years, these engineers have been developing advanced technology for use in medicine. Applications of engineering to medicine range from the development of cryogenic surgical instruments and electronic surveillance systems for hospitals to the design of prototype mechanical hearts. Engineers have devised mathematical models of various parts of the human body in order to better understand how they function. Such analyses include the application of engineering control theory to the function of the human brain and utilization of the principles of fluid mechanics to the study of the blood circulatory system. Moreover, any significant understanding of weight control requires a knowledge of the first law of thermodynamics as applied to humans. In fact, my particular engineering specialties, which are thermodynamics and heat transfer, were, therefore, particularly suited to this area of research.

Many of my friends were openly skeptical. "You can't do that. You can't analyze the human body as if were a machine!" My response was that the human body is a machine. The most complex and challenging machine I had ever analyzed. But I was sure that by taking the proper analytical approach, the weight change equations could be derived.

Developing a Predictive Equation

The analysis method I employed was not new. Engineers call the technique a generalized closed system approach. It has been used to solve many fundamental thermodynamic problems. In simple terms, the analysis is performed by considering the human body as a closed system, and recording what forms of energy and mass cross the system's boundary. Using this method, one is not concerned with what is happening inside the closed system, that is inside the human body. Only external energy and mass transformations are of importance. Once identified these quantities are related in accordance with the conservation of energy. As an analogy, the performance of a large and complex chemical process plant, with its maze of piping and equipment, is routinely understood and predicted by applying the conservation of energy to only the chemical streams entering and leaving the plant – without considering the internal reactions.

In the course of the development and verification of my weight change equations, certain physical, biological, medical and nutritional data were needed. In all cases, I obtained the necessary information from the latest and best available scientific sources.

When finished, my analysis produced the first and only weight change predictive equations in existence at that time. The equations represent a mathematical model of one facet of the human metabolism and provides a means to answer questions such as: How long will it take an individual of a given gender, age, height, weight, and activity level to lose a desired amount of weight when on a known diet? And how should one adjust his/her diet to maintain this lower weight?

Verifying the Equations

Once the weight change equations were derived, the next step was to verify, or validate, that they did indeed accurately predict weight change. There are essentially two ways to accomplish this. The first method involves setting up a series of experiments and observing the weight loss of a number of subjects. This technique would necessitate a research facility and would take years to accomplish. The second method would be to compare the theoretical predictions of my equations against weight loss data gathered over the years by various research teams. Of course, I decided on the latter method.

Although there exists a great deal of weight loss experimental data in the literature, the most famous and comprehensive collection of data was gathered as part of what became known as The Minnesota Experiment. The time-frame was near the end of World War II. A team of research scientists at the Laboratory of Physiological Hygiene at the University of Minnesota had received reports from the U.S. government that starvation was widespread in the occupied countries of Europe and Asia, and in prisoner of war camps. There was a danger of a mass famine. It was apparent that at the end of hostilities the United States would be involved in a large-scale nutritional refeeding program. What was required – urgently – was a project to determine what changes occurred in humans due to semi-starvation and what would be the best sort of rehabilitation diet.

The subjects for the experiment were a volunteer group of U.S. conscientious objectors, who welcomed the opportunity to serve as human guinea pigs. The men were put on diets of approximately 1500 Calories per day for six months. And then they were re-nourished. The data from all phases of the program were recorded in a two-volume treatise entitled *The Biology of Human Starvation*. Among the myriad information gathered during the study was a tremendous amount of carefully documented weight loss data. I analyzed this data and found that my weight loss equation predicted the weight loss experienced by the conscientious objectors quite well.

But I did not stop checking. I compared the predictions of my weight change equation against other well-documented experiments conducted by research laboratories on male and female obese patients. In a variety of tests, patients were subjected to all types of diets – high fat, high protein, low carbohydrate, and so forth. As I suspected, the type of food eaten did not significantly alter my weight loss prediction. For a given subject, only the number of calories consumed appeared to be important. Now satisfied, I wrote a paper documenting my research.

At that time I was employed by IBM and managed an engineering department involved in the design of the first water-cooling system for large computers. Even though I worked on my weight change equations on my own time in the early morning and late at night, the result belonged to IBM. So I had to get IBM's permission to submit for possible publication the paper I called, "The Equations Governing Weight Change in Human Beings." To obtain IBM's permission required that the paper had to pass an internal IBM technical review. But none of the IBM engineers and scientists on the review committee felt they had the background and expertise to judge the paper. But they said they would approve my paper if I obtained the backing of a university professor in the field.

As it happened, I was already in touch with professor Francisco Grande a renowned researcher at the Laboratory of Physiological Hygiene at the University of Minnesota. He had already read my paper and stated that, " ... the paper was a definite contribution to the literature." He later advised me to submit the paper to the *American Journal of Clinical Nutrition*. I didn't realize it at the time that he had been the editor of the AJCN for several years. Needless to say I had no problem getting the paper approved by IBM and then accepted by the AJCN.

A Scientific Paper

"The Equations Governing Weight Change in Human Beings" finally was published in the *American Journal of Clinical Nutrition*. In the paper the disciplines of mathematics, physiology and engineering are merged to establish the foundation for the first truly rational approach to weight control in humans.

A Significant Update

At the time that my weight-loss model was developed, the basil metabolic rate or the energy required to maintain the human body at rest was believed to best be represented by assuming it was dependent on body surface area. But this assumption made the resulting weight loss differential equation non-linear and required a relatively complex numerical solution using programmed software.

Then in 2016, professor of mathematics Diana Thomas at the U.S. Military Academy at West Point suggested that my original model be updated by replacing the resting metabolic rate portion of my model with a much newer, validated and widely used set of regression equations. As a bonus the update also eliminated the non-linearity in my original model and resulted in a differential equation with a much simpler closed-form solution, now called the Antonetti-Thomas weight loss model. This version of the weight loss model was published in 2017 in chapter 12 of the book, *Advances in the Assessment of Dietary Intake* - published by CRC press.

The Weight Control Tables

"Appears quite logical and straightforward," said a chemist friend, after I showed him my original paper. "But," he continued, "it's not going to be used. The average medical doctor or dietician is not sufficiently skilled in math to apply your equations in practical weight control situations. Unless you translate your equations into a more practical form, you've wasted your time!" I realized my friend was right. Even in its simpler updated form, the latest version of my model was still considered too complex to be used by health care professionals. To apply the weight loss equations to a particular individual on a given diet, one would have to be proficient in advanced mathematics. Tables, I thought might be the answer. In tabular form the equations would be useful. Devising a tabular format was almost second nature to me. As a matter of fact, my colleagues at IBM and latter when I was a professor and chair of the mechanical engineering department at

Manhattan College, often would often tease me because of my tendency to arrange virtually any set of data into a table. As you read on you will know what they meant.

In a short time, however, I understood that it would take me years to do the calculations needed to produce the tables I envisioned. It took me almost a half hour to compute just one number in the table and there were thousands of numbers to calculate! But using a computer, calculations of this scope are now commonplace. Luckily I had taught myself how to program early in my engineering career. The resulting tables are published in this book. These unique West Loss Prediction and Weight Maintenance tables make it possible for anyone to quickly determine the exact diet caloric intake needed to lose a given amount of weight in a certain amount of time, or to maintain a desired weight level.

What Is In This Book

In the following chapters, you are introduced to the relationship between weight control and energy. Next is a "cram course" in the basics of sensible nutrition and exercise. Then a new Activity Level Table is introduced and explained. Finally, the heart of the book, the unique Weight Loss Predictive and Weight Maintenance tables are presented. The use of these valuable, innovative tools in the development of a logical and personalized weight control plan is described.

For weight loss, there are 60 unique Weight Loss Prediction tables for men and women. In addition, there are sample 1200 and 1500 kcalorie diets, all with sample no-cooking and cooking daily meal plans complete with delicious recipes.

Use the Weight Loss Prediction tables in conjunction with the Activity Level table, and the sample 1200 and 1500 kcalorie weight loss meal plans to choose the diet calorie level that is best for you. Once you decide on your diet calorie level, you will be directed to NoPaperPress.com where you will find 7-Day, 30-Day, 60-Day, 90-Day and 100-Day (cooking and no-cooking) diets in eBook format.

For weight maintenance, there are 15 Weight Maintenance tables for men and women, and a sample 2500 kcalorie weight maintenance meal plan.

Use the Weight Maintenance tables in conjunction with the Activity Level table, and the sample 2500 kcalorie weight maintenance meal plan to estimate how much you will be able to eat and still maintain your lost weight.

(2500 kcalories is a typical maintenance calorie level for a relatively inactive 45-year-old, 73 kg man). If you want more information, you will be directed to NoPaperPress.com where you will find *Weight Maintenance - Metric Edition*, widely considered the best weight maintenance book available. Finally, the last appendix at the end of this book contains a pertinent Bibliography.

2. Weight and Energetics

All human life depends on energy. Plants convert solar energy into chemical energy by a process called photosynthesis. The chemical energy is then used by plants to make carbohydrates, proteins and fats. We need energy to operate our body, but we cannot use solar energy directly. Instead we get the energy we need from the chemical energy contained in plants or other animals. When we eat food containing carbohydrates, proteins and fats, they are oxidized producing energy, carbon dioxide, water – and heat. This chapter contains a brief discussion of energy, as it generally pertains to our body and how energy relates to weight control.

Conservation of Energy

One of the greatest scientific achievements of the nineteenth century was the recognition and statement of the principle of conservation of energy by Julius Robert Von Mayer, in a classic paper that appeared in 1842 in Liebig's *Annalen der Chemie*. The principle is an inductive generalization based on observation of physical phenomenon and states that energy may be converted or transferred but cannot be created or destroyed. Then in 1847, Von Helmholtz, a surgeon in the Prussian army, wrote a brilliant paper applying the conservation of energy principle to the sciences of physiology and chemistry. By the beginning of the twentieth century, the scientific observations of Rubner, and then Atwater and Benedict, had demonstrated the validity of the law of the conservation of energy for the human metabolism.

According to the law of conservation of energy – as related to humans – the energy value of the food eaten (minus the energy lost in waste) must equal the sum of the heat energy leaving the body plus the physical work done by the body. In weight control, the measure of energy is the Calorie. Both the energy value of the food we eat and the energy we expend in day-to-day activities are expressed in terms of the Calorie. Another way of stating the conservation of energy as related to humans is: Weight is lost when the calories in the food one eats are less than calories one burns in physical activity. This is called a calorie deficit. And the calorie deficit is the driving force for weight loss.

An overwhelming number of scientists today agree that weight change in human beings is linked to their energy balance (or imbalance), and that

weight loss in humans is governed by the law of the conservation of energy.

When Weight Change Occurs

Simply stated, the generally accepted theory is that weight loss in human beings occurs when the energy expended by the body is <u>greater</u> the energy value of the food consumed. When this condition happens an energy imbalance occurs. In order to return to a state of energy balance, the body compensates by "burning" stored body weight, – mainly fat – which results in the liberation of energy. The net effect of this process is a loss of weight and the return of the body to an energy balance or equilibrium, in accord with conservation of energy. Weight gain can be explained by the converse of this reasoning.

Since weight is only lost or gained when there is an energy imbalance, the is no weight change when the energy value of the food eaten equals the amount of energy required by the body to maintain its present weight.

Human Energy Constituents

How much energy does a human being need? To answer this question, one must be aware of the energy constituents that comprise the body's total needs. The energy requirement of an adult human being is made up of three parts:

1. Basal (or resting) Energy: is that energy that is expended performing the body's involuntary basal processes. These processes include circulation, respiration, glandular activity, operation of the kidneys, and contractions of the intestines, etc., all of which consume energy. Scientists determine the basal energy by a carefully controlled test in which measurements are made on a subject that lies quietly and completely relaxed. Test results demonstrate that the basal metabolic energy is dependent on gender, age, height and weight, and that most individuals vary within plus or minus ten percent of what is considered normal.

2. Ingestive Energy: In a classic experiment in calorimetry, the famous French scientist Lavoisier discovered that the ingestion of food caused an increase in the heat produced by the body. This heat increase is due to the physical work involved in the mastication, digestion, and elimination of the food. This process is called the influence of food or specific dynamic action. Ingestive energy was taken into account in deriving the weight control equations and tables in this book.

Another factor which influences the amount of energy expended by humans is the ambient or environmental temperature. But the effect of the ambient temperature is negligible in temperate zones where people are well clothed and homes are well heated.

3. Physical Activity Energy: As soon as one begins to move about, the physical activity causes energy expenditure to increase significantly above the basal level. Many experiments have been performed to determine the energy equivalent of various activities. Test results are usually listed in terms of calories per pound of body weight per unit of time. Thus to compute one's total energy due to physical activity, a diary of the amount of time spent at each activity must be kept for an entire day. The total activity energy would then be calculated by multiplying the amount of time spent at each activity by the caloric value per unit of time for each activity. The activity level for a given individual may be established after measuring the activity energy expended for perhaps ten days and averaging the result.

Activity Levels

Obviously such a determination would in most cases be impractical. Because of this I developed a new and more accessible parameter called the Activity Level. Essentially to use the Activity Level Method, you make a judgment of your physically activity energy expenditure using Table 1 as a guide.

It should be kept in mind that modern technology has, for most people, reduced physical demands, and that most people today are not as active as their ancestors.

- **Average male is between Activity Levels 1 and 2.**
- **Average female probably belongs in Activity Level 1.**

To determine your Activity Level will, in most cases, require considerable judgment on your part. As an aid, Table 1 matches the five Lifestyle Activity Levels to walking distances and an equivalent number of pedometer steps. Choose the option that best approximates the activity of your average day.

Activity Level	Lifestyle	Description	Equivalent Pedometer Steps
0	Sedentary	Inactive most of day. Stands & walks very little during the day.	Less than 3000
1	Relatively Inactive	Seated most of day. Stands & walks at most four hours. Typical of office workers & similar occupations.	About 5000
2	Moderately Active	Stands as often as is seated. Typical of teachers, sales clerks, & similar jobs.	About 8000
3	Very Active	Stands & walks most of day. Typical of factory & construction workers, farmers, & similar jobs.	About 11000
4	Extremely Active	Very hard physical work. Typical of lumber jacks, athletes in training, etc.	17,000 or more

Table 1: Lifestyle Activity Levels

3. Nutrition Basics

Healthy eating habits, the result of sensible nutritional practices, should be an integral part of any weight control program. Foods are made up of seven basic constituents: carbohydrates, proteins, fats, vitamins, minerals, fiber and water. For healthy bodies you need to eat the correct quantity and proportion of all these components. You need protein, carbohydrates and fats, for growth, repair and energy. You need vitamins and minerals, albeit in relatively small quantities, so they can perform their vital roles in the thousands of biochemical reactions in your body. Fiber, the broad name given to the foods you eat that your body cannot digest, but that is needed to assist your digestive system.

Complete & Incomplete Proteins

Proteins are molecules of amino acids that are required for cell maintenance and repair, as well as for the regulation of a wide range of bodily functions. Humans need 22 amino acids in order to live. Our bodies can make 14 of the amino acids on their own, but eight of them, called the essential-amino acids, must be acquired from the foods we eat.

Some foods have all the amino acids needed to build other proteins. These are called complete proteins. Nearly every animal food, including dairy products, eggs, meat, poultry and fish are complete proteins because they contain all eight-essential amino acids. Soy is the only plant-based food that has all eight essential-amino acids.

Other plant-based protein sources lack one or more essential amino acids (i.e., amino acids that the body can not either create, or manufacture by modifying other amino acids.) These **incomplete proteins are found in legumes, grains, nuts, and seeds**. Consuming combinations of foods that have incomplete proteins, however, provide the same complete protein end effect as animal protein. **For a complete-protein meal, simply eat any of the incomplete proteins with another but different incomplete protein**, such as eating legumes with grains, or legumes with nuts or seeds, or grains with nuts or seeds. Examples of some healthy plant-protein combinations (that provide complete protein) are pasta and beans, rice and lentils, corn and beans, bean soup with whole-grain bread, split-pea soup with whole-grain bread, peanut butter on whole-grain bread, and tortillas with refried beans. Note that **proteins contain four calories per gram**.

You Need Healthy Carbs

Carbohydrates provide your body with its basic fuel, the energy your cells need to survive. The staple of most diets around the world, carbohydrates provide essential vitamins and minerals, fiber, and numerous beneficial compounds that promote good health.

Simple carbohydrates, such as sugar, taste sweet, and most are digested and enter your bloodstream quickly. When you eat fruit or drink milk, however, the natural sugar comes with vitamins, minerals (as well as fiber when you eat fruit); whereas the simple sugars in candy, for instance, are nothing but nutritionally-empty calories.

Most complex carbohydrates like nearly all grains (wheat, corn, oats, rice) and foods like potatoes, and pasta generally, but not always, are digested more slowly than simple carbohydrates, and take much longer to enter your bloodstream.

When you eat a sweet food, such as a candy bar, or drink a can of soda, your blood glucose level rises rapidly. In response, your pancreas secretes a large amount of insulin to keep your blood glucose levels from rising too high. The large insulin response in turn tends to cause your blood sugar to fall to levels that are too low. As a consequence, about three to five hours after consuming sweets you feel lethargic and hungry. Many people react to this by eating yet another sweet, which can start a rollercoaster ride of surging glucose and then insulin. None of this is experienced after eating most complex carbohydrates, or after a balanced meal, because the digestion and absorption processes are much slower. Note that **carbohydrates contain four calories per gram**.

Fat Facts

Fats are found in vegetable oil, seeds and nuts, meat and fish, and dairy products, as well as in foods like potato chips and french fries (that are cooked in oil), cookies, cake, and so on. There are certain fats you absolutely need to survive (the essential-fatty acids), and others you would do well to drastically limit (saturated fats) or avoid altogether (trans fats). Chemically all fats have the highest calorie density – containing nine calories per gram.

It is becoming increasingly clear that saturated and trans fats, increase the risk for certain diseases while monounsaturated and polyunsaturated fats, lower the risk. The current scientific thinking regarding fat consumption is as follows:

- **Try to limit the total fat you eat** to no more than 30 percent of your caloric intake.

- **Do not consume foods containing partially-hydrogenated vegetable oil** because they are high in trans fats. This includes commercially prepared baked goods, snack foods, and processed foods, including fast foods. To be on the safe-side, assume these food products contain trans fats unless labeled otherwise.

- **Limit saturated fats**, i.e., any fat of animal origin, to 10 percent of your caloric intake. Have meat less often, and when serving meat use lean cuts and trim the fat. Eat fish and poultry (white meat, without the skin) more frequently. Use fat-free or low-fat-milk dairy products in place of whole-milk dairy products.

- When consuming fat, **choose foods containing monounsaturated fats** like olive oil and canola oil, **and foods rich in polyunsaturated omega-6 and omega-3 fatty acids**.

Try to balance your intake essential fatty acids by eating more omega-3 fatty acids, found in walnuts, tofu, certain seeds and oily fish such as salmon, sardines and tuna.

Fat Type	Where found
Saturated	Meat, poultry (especially the skin), dairy products, lard, coconut oil, palm oil, cocoa butter
Trans Fats	Fried foods, margarine, snack foods, commercially-baked cake and cookies, and fast foods
Cholesterol	Egg yokes, dairy products, organ meats, fatty and prime meats, poultry skin, shellfish (particularly shrimp)
Polyunsaturated (Omega-3)	Mackerel, salmon, sardines, tuna, canola oil, walnuts, flaxseed, wheat germ
Polyunsaturated (Omega-6)	Corn oil, cottonseed oil, safflower oil, sunflower oil, soybean oil
Monounsaturated (Omega-9)	Canola oil, olive oil, safflower oil (hybrid), sunflower oil (hybrid)

Table 2: Fats in Foods

You Need Fiber

Fiber is an important part of a healthy diet. **You need to eat fiber-rich foods to assist your digestive system**. According to the Harvard University School of Public Health, adequate fiber intake reduces the risk of developing various conditions, including heart disease, diabetes, diverticular disease, and constipation.

Three fibers that are eaten on a regular basis are cellulose, hemicellulose and pectin. Hemicellulose is found in the hulls of different grains like wheat; e.g., wheat bran is hemicellulose. Cellulose is the structural component of plants, and gives vegetables their familiar shape. Pectin is found most often in fruits, is soluble in water but non-digestible, and is usually referred to as "water-soluble fiber."

When you eat fiber, in any of its forms, it simply passes straight through, untouched by but aiding your digestive system. Zero calories absorbed!

Vitamins and Minerals

The following is a listing of recommended daily allowance for selected vitamins and minerals. Because this is just a "cram course," the best food source for each of the listed vitamins and minerals is not covered in this book.

Vitamin	Men				Women					
	19-30	31-50	51-70	70+	19-30	31-50	51-70	70+	Preg	Lact
A (mcg)	900	900	900	900	700	700	700	700	770	1300
D (mcg)*	5	5	10	15	5	5	10	15	5	5
E (mcg)	15	15	15	15	15	15	15	15	15	19
K (mcg)*	120	120	120	120	90	90	90	90	90	90
C (mg)	90	90	90	90	75	75	75	75	85	120
B_1 (mg)	1.2	1.2	1.2	1.2	1.1	1.1	1.1	1.1	1.4	1.4
B_2 (mg)	1.3	1.3	1.3	1.3	1.1	1.1	1.1	1.1	1.4	1.6
B_3 (mg)	16	16	16	16	14	14	14	14	18	17
B_5 (mg)*	5	5	5	5	5	5	5	5	6	7
B_6 (mg)	1.3	1.3	1.7	1.7	1.3	1.3	1.5	1.5	1.9	2.0
B_7 (mcg)*	30	30	30	30	30	30	30	30	30	35
B_{12} (mcg)	2.4	2.4	2.4	2.4	2.4	2.4	2.4	2.4	2.6	2.8

Preg = pregnant   Lact = lactating   mcg = micrograms per day   mg = milligrams per day * Values for vitamins D, K, B_5 and B_7 are Adequate Intake because RDAs not established.

Table 3: Recommended Dietary Allowances (RDA) for Selected Vitamins

Mineral	Men				Women					
	19-30	31-50	51-70	70+	19-30	31-50	51-70	70+	Preg	Lact
Calcium (mg)*	1000	1000	1200	1200	1000	1000	1200	1200	1000	1000
Chromium (mcg)*	35	35	30	30	25	25	20	20	30	45
Fluoride (mg)*	4	4	4	4	3	3	3	3	3	3
Iodine (mcg)	150	150	150	150	150	150	150	150	220	290
Iron (mg)	8	8	8	8	18	18	8	8	27	9
Magnesium (mg)	400	420	420	420	310	320	320	320	355	315
Manganese (mg)*	2.3	2.3	2.3	2.3	1.8	1.8	1.8	1.8	2.0	2.6
Molybdenum (mcg)	45	45	45	45	45	45	45	45	50	50
Phosphorus (mg)	700	700	700	700	700	700	700	700	700	700
Potassium (mg)	4700	4700	4700	4700	4700	4700	4700	4700	4700	5100
Selenium (mcg)	55	55	55	55	55	55	55	55	60	70
Zinc (mg)	11	11	11	11	8	8	8	8	8	8

Preg = pregnant, Lact = lactating, mcg = micrograms/day mg = milligrams/day.
*Values for calcium, chromium, fluoride & manganese are Adequate Intake.

Table 4. Recommended Dietary Allowances (RDA) for Selected Minerals

For much more on nutrition including the basic food groups, good food sources for particular vitamins and minerals, phytonutrients, guidelines for healthy eating, vitamin supplements, advice for seniors, how to estimate the calorie content of a meal, calories in foods, etc. see *Eat Smart - Metric Edition* another good book published by NoPaperPress.com.

Eat Slowly

One final important point, try to **eat slowly**. This is especially vital if you are on a diet, trying to lose weight. If you are someone who eats fast, who finishes before everyone else at the table, you are not giving yourself a chance to feel full. While everyone else is still eating, you either sit there and pick, or you have seconds, taking in extra calories you could avoid if you would just slow down. To slow down, try eating smaller mouthfuls, try chewing your food more thoroughly, and try talking more at the table.

4. Exercise Basics

There are two ways to become more physically active: 1) Increase the physical activity in your daily life; and 2) Start on a regular exercise program. Better still would be a combination of both. Here are some ways you can increase physical activity during daily living:

- Change your attitude toward the occasional "bothersome" physical tasks that you encounter in daily living. Consider anytime you have to lift, bend, reach, walk as an opportunity to burn additional calories and as an extension of your formal workout.

- Look for opportunities to walk, such as walking up stairs (two at a time if you can) rather than using an elevator, walking to a local store rather than driving, walking the course if you play golf, and mowing your lawn. At work stand up and stretch at least every two hours, read standing up, etc.

- Engage in leisure activities such as dancing, bowling and gardening as often as you can. They can be enjoyable and provide added exercise.

Each of these daily activities taken alone may not seem like much, but done most days for many years they can add up to a substantial number of extra calories burned.

Select the Right Exercise

Selecting the right fitness exercise is the key to a successful regular conditioning program. You should try to pick an activity (or activities) you will enjoy. Factors to consider in choosing your activity are: your medical condition, your age, your fitness level, your exercise goals, your daily and overall schedule, do you prefer to exercise outdoors or indoors, exercise alone or with others, and how much money you are prepared to spend. You may decide to concentrate on one activity such as squash, or you may choose to walk briskly some days and lift weights on other days. Incidentally, three to five days of a vigorous aerobic exercise plus two days of either strength or flexibility exercises per week is a good combination. Whatever you settle on make sure it is an activity (or activities) that can be done regularly and that you enjoy.

Aerobic Exercise: How Hard?

The central part of your exercise program should be an aerobic (or cardio) exercise done regularly. Additional stretching and strengthening exercises should be included as time allows – but never to the exclusion of the aerobic portion of your program.

An aerobic exercise program should be vigorous enough to condition your cardiovascular system but not so strenuous as to exceed safe limits. Some experts define safe as an exercise pace that is "comfortable." What they mean is that if, for instance, you are jogging or walking briskly you should be able to converse comfortably with a partner and that you should be breathing and feeling normally within ten minutes after you stop exercising. If not, you are exercising too vigorously. Other signs that you are pushing too hard include difficulty breathing, feeling faint, or feeling weak – during or after exercising. If you experience any of these symptoms, you are exercising too intensely and you should cut back.

Activity	Weight (kg)								
	50	**60**	**70**	**80**	**90**	**100**	**110**	**120**	**130**
Aerobics (dance)	450	540	630	720	810	900	990	1080	1170
Basketball	350	420	490	560	630	700	770	840	910
Bicycling (20 kph)	400	479	559	639	719	799	879	959	1039
Cycling	350	420	490	560	630	700	770	840	910
Calisthenics	313	375	438	500	563	625	688	750	813
Cricket	250	300	350	400	450	500	550	600	650
Dancing	229	275	321	366	412	458	504	550	595
Football	376	451	526	602	677	752	827	902	978
Golf (pulling cart)	248	297	347	396	446	495	545	594	644
Golf (riding cart)	174	209	244	278	313	348	383	418	452
Handball	335	402	469	536	603	670	737	804	871
Hiking	294	352	411	470	528	587	646	704	763
Hockey (ice/field)	394	473	552	630	709	788	867	946	1024
Horseback riding	197	236	276	315	355	394	433	473	512
Jogging (12 kph)	624	748	873	998	1122	1247	1372	1496	1621
Raking leaves	301	361	421	482	542	602	662	722	783
Rowing	349	418	488	558	627	697	767	836	906
Sitting	64	77	90	102	115	128	141	154	166
Skating	349	418	488	558	627	697	767	836	906
Skiing (downhill)	303	363	424	484	545	605	666	726	787
Skipping rope	419	503	587	670	754	838	922	1006	1089
Swimming laps	404	484	565	646	726	807	888	968	1049
Tennis (singles)	294	352	411	470	528	587	646	704	763
Tennis (doubles)	223	267	312	356	401	445	490	534	579
Walking (4.8 kph)	178	214	249	285	320	356	392	427	463
Walking (5.5 kph)	218	262	305	349	392	436	480	523	567
Walking (6.5 kph)	277	332	388	443	499	554	609	665	720

Table 5 Caloric Cost (per hour) for Various Activities

If your goal is to burn calories to control your weight and to improve your general health and fitness, walking is a wonderful exercise. Walking does have a downside. Because it is a relatively low-intensity exercise, to get a good workout you have to spend more time walking compared to many other high-intensity exercises.

Get a Pedometer - Count Steps

Sedentary people only take about 2000 to 3000 steps a day. For the average person with a stride equal to about 0,75 meter, 1320 steps amounts to walking about one kilometer.

A Harvard University study has shown that 6000 steps a day correlate with lower death rates in men, and that 8000 to 10000 step per day promote weight loss. And these health and weight management benefits don't oblige you to walk continuously until you accrue the required number of steps. Rather, all steps throughout the day to wherever and whenever count toward your daily total.

Strength-Building Programs

As good as aerobic exercises are, they contribute little to building upper-body strength. If you are a beginner interested in strength training it's probably worthwhile to start by joining a health club, where you can get professional instruction on the proper use of exercise equipment, from dumbbells to rowing machines, and where you can compare different exercise routines and develop a personalized fitness program.

Of all the many strength-building options, I personally prefer free weights (actually dumbbells) because they can be used at home. Working out at home has some significant advantages. First, your workout takes less time because you don't have to drive back and forth to a health club; second, you have the flexibility of dividing your workout into small time segments to fit your day, whenever you have time, such as when the baby is napping, and of course working out at home is certainly less expensive.

You can workout in a bedroom, basement, garage, attic – anywhere you have extra space. A set of variable (adjustable) weight dumbbells and a small weight bench don't take up much room and are all you need for a home-based gym. Choose dumbbell exercises that comprise a total-body workout, that are suitable for beginners, and that involve all the major muscle groups. Bear in mind, **knowledge and the discipline to work out regularly are far more important than fancy equipment.**

Risks and Possible Problems

Certain situations may occur that indicate you may be doing too much, exercising too hard. For example, regardless of your pulse rate you should never be left completely breathless by your aerobic exercise. A good rule to remember is: **You are exercising too hard if you cannot carry on a**

conversation while you are jogging, cycling, etc. A feeling of having worked hard is fine, sweating is good, but not a feeling of undo fatigue.

Perhaps the most frequent problems faced by exercisers are injuries of the joints and muscles: sprains and strains, knee pain, elbow pain, back pain, neck pain, shin splints and stress fractures. Most happen when you exercise too hard.

Potentially serious problems are signaled if you experience any of the following symptoms during or after exercise. The symptoms include but are not limited to any abnormal heart action, such as an irregular heart rhythm, pain or pressure in the middle of your chest, pain in an arm or your neck, dizziness, fainting or lightheadedness, severe exhaustion, sudden loss of coordination, or confusion. If any of these symptoms are experienced, stop exercising immediately and get medical help.

Avoiding Injury

My good friend and frequent workout buddy, A.C. Kanaar, M.D., specialized in rehabilitation medicine but he also preached what he called "preventive medicine," that is avoiding injury by practicing a common-sense approach to exercise:

- Have a medical checkup and then set realistic fitness goals.
- Build up your exercise intensity gradually over many weeks, months.
- After you eat a meal, wait about two hours before exercising.
- Buy good equipment suitable for your exercise routine.
- Use safety and protective equipment when appropriate, such as helmet when you bicycle, and goggles when you play handball, squash or racquetball.
- Do not exercise on very hot day or very cold days.
- If you insist on working out in very hot or cold weather, always let someone know when and where you will be exercising and when you are planning to return.
- If you are new to a gym or health club, attend an orientation session before you use any unfamiliar exercise equipment. Otherwise, read the operating instructions carefully, and ask someone qualified for help.
- For aerobic activities, warm up slowly and cool down slowly after you exercise.

- Do not increase the difficulty of any activity (e.g., your walking or jogging distance, the amount of weight you lift) by more than 10 percent per week.
- Jog on softer surfaces such as a level grass field, a dirt path, or a running track.
- After exercising wait 30 minutes before eating.
- As a final point, if you experience some early warning pain stop exercising.

Control Your Weight & Stay Healthy

Remember it doesn't matter exactly what exercises you choose, what equipment you use, or what facility you use. These are secondary factors. What matters most is that you exercise consistently. **To improve muscle tone and overall fitness, feel good and stay healthy, you should exercise at least five days per week, day after day, week after week, year after year – for as long as you are physically able.** Remember the key words: consistent, determined, steady, persistent, dogged, unswerving, gritty, single-minded. Consistent!

For much more on exercise I recommend *Exercise **Smart - U.S. Edition***, another excellent book published by NoPaperPress.

5. About Your Weight

Why are you overweight? Once you accept the fact that your weight is governed by the conservation of energy, the answer is simple enough. You are overweight because you consume more calories than you expend. Overeating or inactivity, or a combination of both, are the culprits. But they are the cause of your overweight, not the reason for it.

The question might more properly be: Why do you eat more than you should? The popular notion that most people are overweight or obese because of a defect in their metabolism is just not supported by scientific evidence. In fact, being overweight or obese most often can be attributed to how we adapt to our 21st century environment and to our heredity. More specifically, the major causes of obesity and overweight are as follows:

- **Environmental**: We live in a society where food is abundant and where strenuous physical activity is, for most people, a thing of the past. In other words, we eat too much and do too little. This is by far the most important factor.

- **Genetic**: Everyone starts life with a different body type. Researchers agree there is a relationship between the body type we inherit and the likelihood and ease with which we become overweight. Three basic body types are illustrated in the figure on the next page. The active ectomorph, with a typically long, narrow body and light appetite will find it difficult indeed to gain weight or to become overweight. On the other extreme, the more sedentary endomorph with a hearty appetite faces a life-long struggle against obesity. Depending on their appetite and how active they are, even muscular mesomorphs often gain unwanted weight as they age. Because everyone has some features of each body type, we are all born with different weight gaining tendencies.

- **Psychological**: There are a great many people who overeat and become overweight in response to tension, frustration, or other psychological issues.

- **Developmental**: Early forced feeding often leads to childhood-onset obesity. Overeating then becomes habitual and an excessive number of fat cells are formed early on that are difficult to shed later in life.

- **Metabolic and Regulatory**: Sometimes overeating is caused by a damaged hypothalamus or an incorrect interpretation of the hunger/satiety signal. Though relatively rare, a defect in the thyroid or pituitary gland can also cause a change in metabolic rate. All can result in overweight. I am going to assume that you have consulted with your physician and have no physiological disorder (glandular, digestive, etc.) that would prevent you from losing weight. Very few people are overweight because of this sort of ailment.

The fact is that although you may never understand the underlying cause for your being overweight, you still can do something about it. You can still lose weight successfully by understanding and applying the basics of sound diet theory.

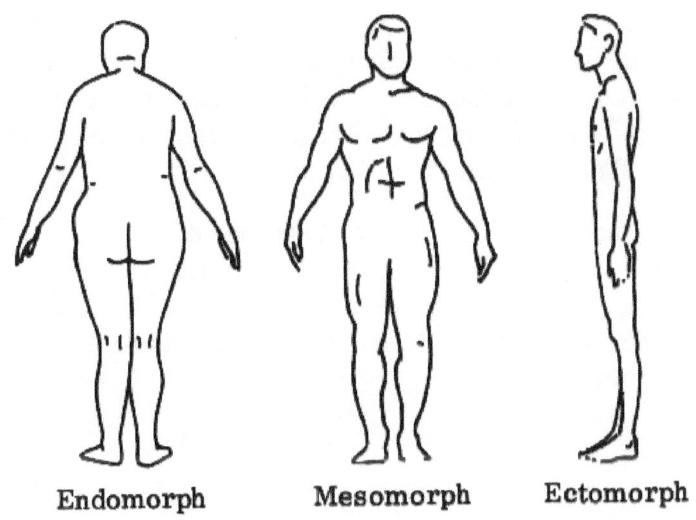

Human Body Types

What You Should Weigh

Body Weight Mass Index, or BMI is currently the method used by physicians and researchers to assess a person's weight. To utilize the common place BMI chart, one enters the chart with their height and weight and determines their BMI. Then another chart is used to convert the BMI into a weight profile.

I devised a more convenient way, that is to use a New BMI-Based Weight vs. Height Chart shown in Table 6, where the underweight category corresponds to BMI = 18.5 or less, normal weight is for BMI = 18.6 to 24.9, overweight is for BMI = 25.0 to 29.9, obese is for BMI = 30.0 to 39.9 and extremely obese

is for BMI = 40 or more. Readers should strive to get their BMI into the normal category, or 18.6 to 24.9.

Body Fat Percentage

Many health care professionals contend that overweight or obesity does not depend on body weight but on the amount of body fat a person carries compared to their total body weight.

Body fat exists in two storage sites. The first storage depot, consists of the intestines, muscles, and the lipid-rich tissues throughout the central nervous system. This is referred to as Essential Fat and is required, or essential to maintain health. In females, essential fat also includes sex-specific or sex-characteristic fat. The average woman requires approximately 10% essential fat, and the average man about 3%. The higher percentage of essential fat in females includes about 7% of sex-specific fat, believed to be important for child-bearing and other hormone-related functions.

This is an important topic but is beyond the scope of this book. For more information, including the following new unique tables: Body Fat Percentage, Maximum Waist Size, Optimum Waist Size, Waist to Hip Ratio, see ***Professional Weight Control - Metric Edition*** an eBook also published by NoPaperPress.com.

Height (cm)	Normal Weight (kg)	Overweight (kg)	Obese (kg)
150	42 – 56	57 – 67	68 – 90
153	44 – 58	59 – 70	71 – 93
156	46 – 61	62 – 73	74 – 97
159	48 – 63	64 – 76	77 – 101
162	50 – 65	66 – 79	80 – 105
165	51 – 68	69 – 81	82 – 109
168	53 – 70	71 – 84	85 – 113
171	55 – 73	74 – 87	88 – 117
174	57 – 75	76 – 90	91 – 121
177	59 – 78	79 – 94	95 – 125
180	61 – 81	82 – 97	98 – 129
183	63 – 83	84 – 100	101 – 134
186	65 – 86	87 – 103	104 – 138
189	67 – 89	90 – 107	108 – 143

Table 6: New BMI-Based Weight vs. Height

6. Weight Loss

In the short term only, the energy value of weight change is approximately 3500 Calories for one pound of weight lost or gained. But for longer duration diets with more weight loss, this rule does not apply. In most practical diet situations, the Weight Loss Prediction model I developed, or the Weight Loss Prediction Tables must be used.

Diet Options

Once you have utilized **Table 1** on page 18 to settle on your Activity Level, you are ready to use the Weight Loss Prediction tables, to determine your diet calorie options. Weight Loss Prediction Tables are located in **Appendix A for men** (page 54) and in **Appendix B for women** (page 91), and are organized by gender, age, height, weight and activity level. Use of the tables is best illustrated by an example.

<u>Example 1</u>: A 28-year-old woman, who is 1.56 meters tall and weighs 70 kilograms, has essentially a sedentary job as a computer programmer and spends most of her free time in front of a TV set. How long will it take her to lose 8 kilos?

Considering her job and leisure-time pursuits, from Table 1, she decides she is Activity Level 1. Next she consults Appendix B and finds the Weight Loss Prediction table that applies to her is **Table B.1** (page 92), labeled "Weight Loss Prediction: Women 18 to 35 yrs, 150 to 165 cm, Activity Level 1." Table 7, below, shows a portion of Table B.1.

Height: 150 to 165 cm   Activity Level 1

Weight Loss	Diet kcalories	Present Weight (kg.)							
		50	55	60	65	70	80	90	100
2	900	17	15	14	13	[illegible]	11	9	9
2	1200	25	21	19	17	[illegible]	13	11	10
2	1500	43	34	28	24	[illegible]	17	14	12
2	1800	178	82	54	41	[illegible]	24	19	15
4	900	35	31	29	26	[illegible]	21	19	17
4	1200	51	44	38	34	[illegible]	26	23	20
4	1500	92	70	58	49	[illegible]	34	29	25
4	1800		186	117	86	[illegible]	49	38	31
6	900		48	44	40	[illegible]	32	29	26
6	1200		67	59	52	[illegible]	40	35	31
6	1500		111	90	76	[illegible]	52	44	37
6	1800			191	136	[illegible]	75	58	48
8	900		66	60	54	50	44	39	35
8	1200		93	81	72	64	54	47	41
8	1500		157	125	[illegible]	90	71	59	51
8	1800			283	194	149	103	80	65
10	900			76	69	64	55	49	44
10	1200			104	92	82	69	59	52
10	1500			164	135	116	91	75	64

Table 7: Portion of Table B.1 (Illustrates Example 1)

To use the portion of Table B.1 shown above, our dieter would scan the far left of the table and locates her desired weight loss of 8 kilos. She finds four different diet options of 900, 1200, 1500 and 1800 kcalories. From this point, she runs a finger horizontally (to the right) until it intersects the vertical column headed by her present weight of 70 kilograms. The four numbers in the box at the intersection are the time in days to lose 8 kilos, depending on the diet kcalories consumed. Specifically, to lose 8 kilos our fictional female's diet kcalorie options are:

- 900 kcalories per day for 50 days.
- 1200 kcalories per day for 64 days.
- 1500 kcalories per day for 90 days.
- 1800 kcalories per day for 149 days.

Which alternative should she choose? Many health-care professionals recommend a gradual weight loss of one kilo per week. The reason for the relatively slow weight loss is that you want to be on the diet long enough to understand and learn how much to eat, and how to eat properly. In this case, at one kilo per week her diet should last 8 weeks or 56 days, and at one-half kilo per week her diet should take 16 weeks or 112 days.

To comply with accepted weight loss guidelines, therefore, she should choose a diet calorie level that will result in her losing the 8 kilos over a 56 to 112 day period - pointing to the 1200 or 1500-kcalorie options. In the end, it comes down to deciding between the shorter term 1200-kcalorie diet or a longer duration somewhat higher 1500-kcalorie option.

Better still would be for this woman to increase her activity level by taking a brisk five-kilometer walk everyday, and qualifying for Activity Level 2, the moderately active category and (**Table B.2** on page 93) which would result in the following shorter-duration diet options:

- 900 kcalories per day for 43 days.
- 1200 kcalories per day for 53 days.
- 1500 kcalories per day for 69 days.
- 1800 kcalories per day for 99 days.

Hence, by increasing her activity level, she could decrease the time to lose the 8 kilos by 14 to 32 percent – depending on the diet-calorie level she chooses.

Suppose Your Weight Isn't In Table?

Suppose the woman in Example 6.1 weighed 75 kilograms and wanted to lose 8 kilos on a 1500-kcalorie Diet. But 75 kilos is not listed in Table B.1. However, by noting that the time required to lose 8 kilos when weighing 75 kilos would be half-way between the times shown in the table for 70 and 80 kilos, she would proceed as follows. First, from Table B.1, she would find that that at 70 kilos it would take her 91 days to lose 8 kilos, and at 80 kilos it would take 71 days. The time on a diet at 75 kilos would be in the middle of these two, or about 80 days. This estimating technique is called interpolation and should be used whenever you can't find your exact weight in one of the tables.

If math was never your strong suit, don't give up! Get a friend to help. The important part – the doing – comes after the calculations. That's where you come in.

The Physiology of Weight Loss

Weight lost during periods of negative energy balance is of variable composition. Fat, water, and protein are lost at different rates and at different stages of a reducing diet. The amount of water in humans also varies from day to day. Over reasonable period of time, however, the amount of water entering the body will equal the amount leaving. And the water balance of the body is then said to be in equilibrium.

A considerable loss of water usually occurs at the start of a diet. Because a pint of water weighs about one pound, this initial water loss will appear as a weight loss. But the weight loss is not "real," because no body tissue has been lost. (From this point on, when reference is made to "real" weight loss, what is meant is that weight loss which will not be regained, once the body's water balance is restored.)

Many theories have been proposed to explain this phenomenon but none have been confirmed scientifically. Because of changes in body hydration, you will usually notice higher weight loss during the first week or two on a diet than the Weight Loss Prediction Tables forecast. By the following week, however, the water balance of the body will readjust and your weight loss will more closely approach the values in the Weight Loss Prediction Tables. The tables predict "real" weight loss. In addition, realize that the weight of a normal person fluctuates two to three pounds daily. Your weight is lowest before breakfast and highest in the evening before retiring. So to determine your weight loss, always weigh yourself at the same time of day.

In women, another cause of weight fluctuation is water retention just prior to their menstrual period. This is not uncommon and may appear to be a time when weight is not lost. Again, by the next week, the water balance of the body will readjust and your weight loss will more closely approach the values in the Weight Loss Prediction Tables.

Weight Loss Principles

Once the parameters involved in weight loss are related in a mathematical equation, it is possible to state some principles. (It is also possible to deduce the following truisms by examining the Weight Loss Prediction tables.)

- Given two people the same age, gender and activity level, and on the same reducing diet, **the heavier person will lose weight faster than the thinner person**. For instance, according to **Table A.1** (page 55) on 1500 kcalories, it would take a 25-year old, 160 cm, 60-kg male (Activity Level 1) 46 days to lose 4 kilos; whereas the same table indicates a 120-kg male would only take only 17 days to lose 4 kilos – less than half the time!

- Given two people the same age, gender and activity level, and on the same reducing diet (i.e., consuming the same number of calories), the **taller person will lose weight at a faster rate**.

- Given a male and female, the same age, weight, activity level and on the same reducing diet, **the man will lose weight faster than the woman**. This is due to the fact that women have lower basal metabolic rates than men and therefore must eat less than a man to lose the same amount of weight.

- Given two individuals, the same gender, weight and activity level, **the younger person will lose weight much faster than the older person.** The lesson is if you are overweight start on a weight loss diet now because it will only become **more difficult to lose weight as you get older.**

- It follows that if your **caloric intake is constant over the years you will slowly gain weight as you age.** This is because your basal metabolic rate decreases as you advance in age, and most people tend not to be as active as they get older.

Selecting a Weight Loss Diet

As mentioned previously, this book does not actually contain a diet. But there are sample 1200 and 1500 kcal **nutritionally balanced diets** (see **Chapter 8** on page 47), all with sample no-cooking and cooking daily meal plans complete with a delicious recipe.

The sample diets give you an idea of how much food you can eat at a given calorie level. Of course, on a 900 kcal diet you would be eating 300 kcal less than on the 1200 kcal diet, and on an 1800 kcal diet you would have 300 kcal more to eat than on a 1500 kcal diet.

Incidentally, a 900 kcal diet is usually not recommended. This is because it is difficult to obtain all the nutrients you need on 900 Calories, and it is also difficult to stay on a very low calorie diet over the long term.

Use the weight loss prediction tables in conjunction with the activity level table, and then the sample 1200 and 1500 kcal weight loss daily meal plans to help you select the diet calorie level that is best for you. Only 1200 and 1500 kcal meal plans are shown here, but be aware that 900 and 1800 kcal plans are also available in some NoPaperPress eBooks.

Once you decide on your diet calorie level, you can navigate to NoPaperPress.com for complete 7-Day, 30-Day and 60-Day diets - both cooking and no-cooking. Incidentally, **no-cooking diet books are unique to NoPaperPress.**

7. Weight Maintenance

Most people can lose weight on almost any diet, but the crucial issue is whether the weight loss can be maintained. The real challenge is not losing weight but keeping it off! Few, if any, of the popular weight control programs have been successful at maintaining weight over the long term. There are two key concerns with respect to weight maintenance:

1. **Preventing people from gaining weight as they age**.

2. **Preventing the regaining of lost weight, i.e., helping people keep off weight they've lost**.

In fact both of these vexing issues can be approached and solved using virtually the same weight control techniques. First you need to understand why you gain or regain weight.

Why You Gain Weight With Age

A study, published in a 2005 issue of the Annals of Internal Medicine, that followed 4000 adults for three decades suggests that in the long term, 90 percent of men and 70 percent of women will become overweight (with a BMI $\geq$ 25). Interestingly, half of the men and women in the study, who had made it well into adulthood without a weight problem, ultimately also became overweight and a third became obese (BMI $\geq$ 30).

Why does this happen? When you reach your mid to late twenties, you slowly start to lose muscle and add fat as part of the natural aging process. As you age your muscle mass slowly deteriorates and is replaced by fat. But muscle is active tissue and requires lots of energy (calories) for growth and repair; whereas, fat is basically inactive and uses very few calories to exist. So as you age and you lose muscle mass your metabolism gradually slows. In fact your metabolism decreases about 10 percent every decade. If you are like the average adult, at some point, because of your slowing metabolism, you could start to gain almost one kilo every year. To offset this, you need to cut back on calories, or increase your physical activity, or both. Otherwise the excess calories will add up and so will your weight! The point being that you can never become complacent. **You must continually watch your weight because we are all at risk of becoming overweight.**

Why You Gain Weight After a Diet

After any diet, your lower body weight requires fewer calories to function. In other words, your lower body weight results in a slower overall metabolism.

Within five years, most dieters regain every pound they have lost. Why? In most cases it's because after losing weight most people eventually revert to their pre-diet eating and exercising habits, and this inevitably leads to their regaining the weight they lost – and often more. The fact is **the less you weigh, the less you need to eat to maintain your lower weight**.

Without some lifestyle modifications, if you are like the average adult you will regain every pound you have lost. It's a fact that 95 percent of dieters, that's 95 out of 100 people, regain all the weight they lost and often more!

People Who Regained Lost Weight

A study published in the American Journal of Preventive Medicine, surveyed about 1300 adults from the 1999 to 2002 who were overweight or obese and had lost at least 10 percent of their maximum weight. The study authors found some common characteristics associated with those who regained lost weight:

- They spent four hours or more per day in front of a TV set or computer.
- They lost a lot of weight (at least 20% of their max. weight) in a short time.
- They started regaining lost weight soon after they stopped dieting.

Most of the above make sense. Too much TV or computer time usually means these people were undoubtedly sedentary and less likely to get lots of exercise.

Losing weight too fast, either by fad or extreme dieting, can leave people feeling deprived and often ends up triggering binges that go on until the lost weight is regained.

It takes time to establish a new lifestyle that supports weight maintenance. People who have lost weight and then quickly gained it back, may not have had the time to acquire all the skills needed to maintain their lower weight.

People Who Maintained Lost Weight

The National Weight Control Registry studied people who had lost at least 30 pounds and kept it off for more than a year. What they found was that

although people lost weight differently, they kept it off similarly. Here are some common traits of the successful maintainers:

- Most maintainers ate a low-fat diet - but not a hugely restrictive one.
- All successful maintainers monitor their portion sizes.

- Nearly four in five eat breakfast every day.
- Most are physically active, with walking their most common activity.
- They walk for nearly an hour every day.
- They weighed themselves once a week.
- These people probably were not spending four plus hours watching TV.
- They found pleasure in their healthier lifestyle and freedom from constant dieting.

Select Correct Weight Maintenance Table

The Weight Maintenance Calorie tables display how many the calories you can eat without gaining or losing weight. Or put another way how many calories you can consume and not regain your lost weight.

First, you need to select the Weight Maintenance Table that's right for you. The tables are organized by gender, age, height, weight and activity level. In this book you will find an updated set of 15 Weight Maintenance tables in **Appendix C for men** (page 116) and in **Appendix D for women** (page 126).

How to Use the Weight Maintenance Tables

Use of the Weight Maintenance Tables is best illustrated by the following example.

Example 2: Consider a 53-year-old relatively inactive (Activity Level 1), 170 cm tall, female who weighed 90 kg at the start of her reducing diet. After losing 20 kg, she weighed 70 kg. Determine her weight maintenance calories before and after she lost weight.

From **Table D.4** (on page 130) she finds that before she started her diet, when she weighed 90 kg, 2726 kcalories, meaning she must have been eating about 2726 kcalories of food per day. After her diet, the same table shows that in order to maintain her lower weight of 70 kg she must restrict her food intake in the future to 2336 kcalories per day. On average then, to neither gain nor lose weight at 70 kg she must consume about 2726 − 2336 = 390 kcalories per day less than she did when she weighed 90 kg.

This person could help her cause by engaging in some form of exercise everyday. For example, if she walked 45 minutes every day at moderate 5.5 kph pace (covering a distance of slightly more than 4 kilometers), she could eat an additional (305 − 90) x 45/60 = 161 kcal per day without gaining weight.

Incidentally, for readers who have lost weight and want to keep it off, or for those who don't want to gain weight as they age, I recommend a book I recently wrote, the only ebook devoted to entirely to weight maintenance, called *Weight Maintenance - Metric Edition* again published by NoPaperPress. com.

Weight Maintenance is a Life-Long Struggle

A trim 43 year-old nutritionist laughs when people say, "Oh, you're so lucky to be naturally thin." Her reply, "Give me break. I workout and do you think I eat everything I want?"

Staying lean requires constant vigilance. In weight maintenance, it is the number of calories you eat over the long term that is important. As an illustration, the weight maintenance value of 2336 kcal per day for the 53-year-old woman in Example 2 amounts to about 878000 kcal in a single year. Now realize that an annual error of only two percent of this total (that is roughly 17600 kcal per year, or 48 kcal per day) would result in a weight gain of (17600 kcal / 7700 kcal per kg = 2.3 kg) more than two kilos in one year, and the importance of knowing and adhering to your personal weight maintenance calorie value becomes apparent. In brief, **to control your weight it is the number of calories eaten over the long term that matters**.

Obviously, it would be impossible for the woman in Example 2 to eat exactly 2297 kcal day after day. Errors are inevitable and experience has shown that when people err they do so on the high side. They consume more calories than their maintenance value, rarely less. To allow for occasional overeating or days when don't have time to exercise, it is recommended that you plan to eat about seven percent below the values in the weight maintenance tables. For the female in Example 2, that would mean about 2140 kcal per day rather than the 2297 kcal shown in her Weight Maintenance table – leaving her room for an occasional calorie splurge, or a missed exercise session.

Get Off the Diet Roller Coaster

For most people, a shape-up program consists of getting on the latest diet bandwagon. But short-term diets are temporary and rarely work. It makes no sense to go on a diet for a few months, only to regain the weight. Losing weight is comparatively easy; the challenging part is keeping it off. Instead of short-term fixes, you should focus on developing better eating and exercise habits – that you can stay with over the long haul. Instead of going on and off diets, you should change your approach and make exercise and good nutrition a way of life.

Get off the diet roller coaster once and for all by developing habits that you will be able to maintain for the rest of your life. It may take a little more discipline, patience and hard work this way, but it the end it will all be worth it. To lose weight permanently, you must make a commitment to a healthier way of life. So get started.

8. Sample Weight Loss & Maintenance Diets

In this chapter you will be introduced to 1200 and 1500 kcal sample weight loss diets and a 2500 kcal weight maintenance meal plan. The purpose of these sample diets is to help you appreciate how much food you can eat at these calorie levels.

Weight Loss: 1200 and 1500 kcal diets are most often recommended by health care professionals. Use the 1200 and 1500 kcal sample diets to understand how much food you can eat at these calorie levels. If after referring the Weight Loss Prediction tables, you are considering a 900 kcal diet just subtract 300 kcal worth of food from the sample 1200 kcal diet. In the same manner, if you think an 1800 kcal diet would be right for you, add 300 kcal of food to the 1500 kcal sample diet.

Weight Maintenance: After using the Weight Maintenance tables to determine the appropriate calorie level for your new lower weight, add or subtract calories from the sample 2500 kcal weight maintenance meal plan to understand how much food you can eat without regaining your lost weight.

The 1200 and 1500 kcal diets and the 2500 kcal weight maintenance meal plan are from the following NoPaperPress eBooks and are reprinted with the permission of NoPaperPress.com.

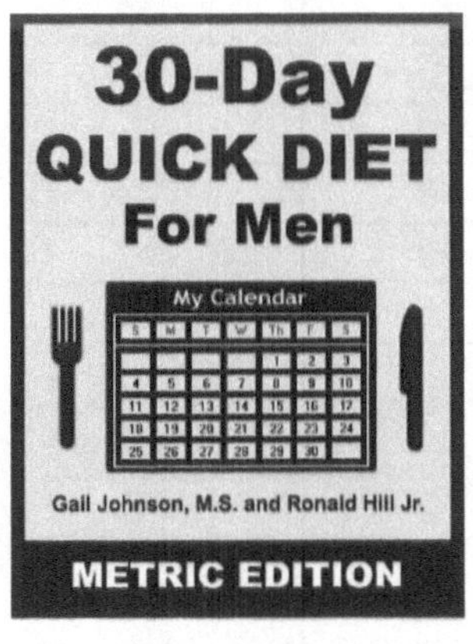

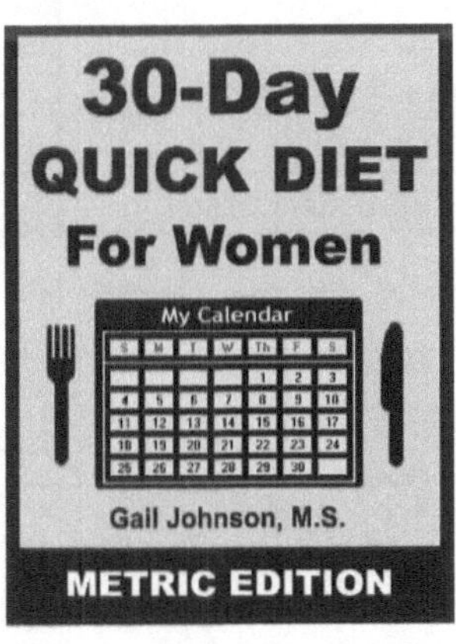

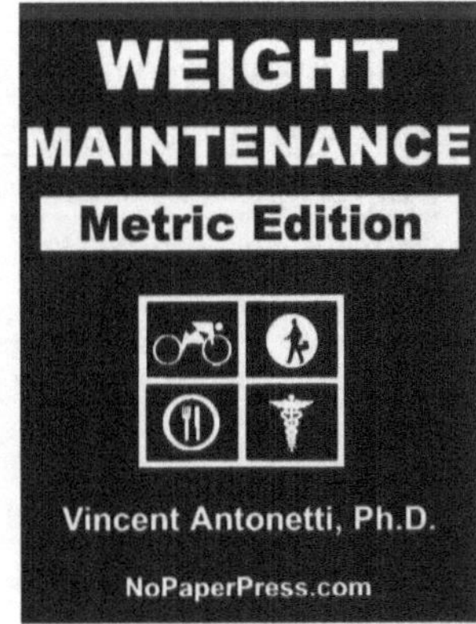

Table 8. Sample 1200 Calorie Meal Plan

Day 2   1200 Calorie Diet

BREAKFAST	Calories	Totals
Orange juice (120 ml)	50	
Wheaties (30 g) + 120 ml skim milk + ½	190	
Coffee	10	250 kcal
SNACK		
Fresh fruit in season (apple, pear, etc)	70	
Coffee or tea	10	80 kcal
LUNCH		
Vegetable soup (240 ml)	110	
Turkey breast (30 g) on 1 slice rye bread	105	
Pickle spears	0	
Lettuce & tomato slices	20	
Hot or iced tea	10	245 Cal
SNACK		
Popcorn Mini bag	110	
Coffee or tea	10	120 kcal
DINNER		
Baked Herb-Crusted Cod (Day 2 Recipe)	230	
Spinach (75 g) steamed with garlic &	70	
Asparagus (7 spears cooked & drained)	20	
Whole-grain bread (1 slice)	70	
Water with lemon wedge	10	400 kcal
SNACK		
Crackers or biscuits – any brand	90	
Coffee or tea	10	100 kcal
		1200 Cal

Table from: ***30-Day Quick Diet for Women - Metric Edition*** with permission of NoPaperPress.com.

Day 2 - Recipe

Baked Herb-Crusted Cod

 4 Cod fish fillets – 120 to 150 g each
 2 tablespoons (Tbsp) flour (50 g)
 2 Tbsp cornmeal (50 g)
 2 Tbsp minced fresh herbs
 2 teaspoons (tsp) lemon juice (10 ml)

Sprinkle cod with lemon juice. Mix flour, cornmeal and herbs and dust the cod with the cornmeal- herb mixture. Bake in oven at 190 °C for 10 minutes. Add salt and black pepper to taste.

Serves 4. One serving is about 230 kcal (for cod only).

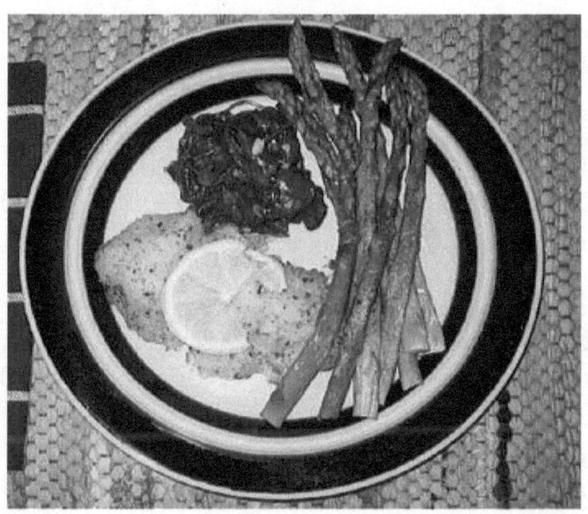

Diet Tip of the Day: When you're on a diet, eating in a restaurant can be a challenge, because most restaurant portions are huge, and can easily total more than 1000 kcal. So, in a restaurant decide how much to eat – and take the remainder home. A good general rule is to **eat half and bring the remainder home**.

Recipe from: ***30-Day Quick Diet for Women - Metric Edition*** with permission of NoPaperPress.com.

Table 9: Sample 1500 Calorie Meal Plan

BREAKFAST	kcal	Totals
Grapefruit (½ medium size)	75	
Cheerios (30 g) + 120 ml skim milk + 15 raisins	190	
Coffee	10	275 kcal
MORNING SNACK		
Fresh fruit in season (apple, peach, plum, etc)	70	
Coffee or tea	10	80 kcal
MID-DAY MEAL		
Cottage cheese – low fat (225 g)	180	
Large tossed salad with 30 ml low-cal dressing	70	
Small whole-grain roll	80	
Hot or ice tea	10	340 kcal
AFTERNOON SNACK		
Handful of unsalted mixed nuts	100	
Coffee or tea	10	110 kcal
EVENING MEAL		
Grilled swordfish (Day 18 Recipe)	250	
Grilled potatoes	100	
Grilled cherry tomatoes	45	
Spinach (75 g) steamed & drizzled 5 ml olive il	70	
Whole-grain bread (1 slice)	65	
Water with lemon section	0	530 kcal
EVENING SNACK		
Two small chocolate chip cookies – or	160	
Coffee or tea	10	170 kcal
		1505

Table from: ***30-Day Quick Diet for Men- Metric Edition*** with permission of NoPaperPress.com.

Day 18 - Recipe

Grilled Swordfish with Citrus-Herb Marinade

550 g swordfish
1 bottle citrus-herb marinade
24 cherry tomatoes
4 medium potatoes
250 g fresh spinach
1 pinch rosemary & juice of ¼ lemon
10 ml extra-virgin olive oil

Steam spinach with garlic and drizzle with olive oil.
Cut up potatoes and place sprinkle with lemon juice, add rosemary, salt and black pepper. Place on grill for about 10 minutes, turning occasionally.
Toss cherry tomatoes in small amount olive oil. Add fresh oregano, salt and black pepper. Place on heavy-duty aluminum foil, seal and grill for about 3 minutes.
Marinade swordfish in citrus-herb vinaigrette. Grill on hot fire for about 5 minutes on one side and 3 minutes on the other, or until done as desired.
<u>Serves 4</u>. One plate consisting of grilled swordfish (250 kcal) with grilled potatoes (100 kcal) and cherry tomatoes (45 kcal) and steamed spinach (50 kcal) totals 445 kcal.

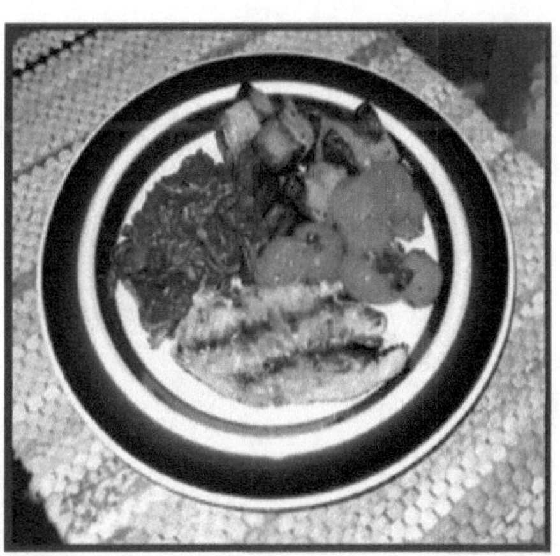

<u>Diet Tip of the Day:</u> Do not be in a hurry to lose weight. Slower weight loss is healthier, is more likely to be permanent, and is easier to sustain over the long haul.

Recipe from: ***30-DayQuck Diet For Men - Metric Edition*** with permission of NoPaperPress.com.

Table 10: Sample Weight Maintenance Meal Plan

BREAKFAST	Calories	Totals
Grapefruit (½)	75	
Fried eggs (2 eggs)	200	
Turkey bacon (2 slices)	70	
Whole wheat toast (2 slices with butter)	250	
Coffee	10	605 kcal
MORNING SNACK		
Yogurt (170 g nonfat, any flavor)	100	
Coffee or tea	10	110 kcal
LUNCH		
Ham (85 g) w mustard on 2 slices bread	370	
Lettuce & tomato slices	20	
Vegetable soup (200 ml)	100	
Fresh fruit in season (apple, peach, plum, etc)	70	
Hot or iced tea	10	570 kcal
AFTERNOON SNACK		
Large handful of mixed nuts	150	
Coffee or tea	10	160 kcal
DINNER		
Chicken with Peppers & Onions (See Recipe)	250	
Sautéed red peppers with onions	70	
Green beans - steamed	25	
Mashed cauliflower	30	
Large tossed green salad with 30 ml dressing	200	
Whole-grain bread (1 slice)	65	
Glass of red wine (175 ml)	150	
Water with lemon wedge	15	805 kcal
EVENING SNACK		
Three small cookies	240	
Coffee or tea	10	250 kcal
		2500

Table adapted from: ***Weight Maintenance - Metric. Edition*** with permission of
NoPaperPress.com.

Sample - Weight Maintenance Recipe

Chicken with Peppers & Onions

4   boneless & skinless chicken breasts (about 140 g each)

Coat the chicken breasts in a bottled barbeque sauce. Prepare medium-hot fire on well-oiled gas or charcoal grill. Place breasts on grill, turning them every 4 minutes, for 10 to 12 minutes, or until done. (To check if breasts are done, the meat should be moist and white with no sign of pink when you cut into breast.) Serve hot.

2   medium red peppers
1   medium onion

Place peppers and onions in pan with 30 ml fat-free chicken stock. Sauté until stock is reduced. Spray pan lightly with non-stick cooking oil and sauté another 2 minutes. Salt and pepper to taste.

Serves 4. About 250 kcal per serving (for chicken only).

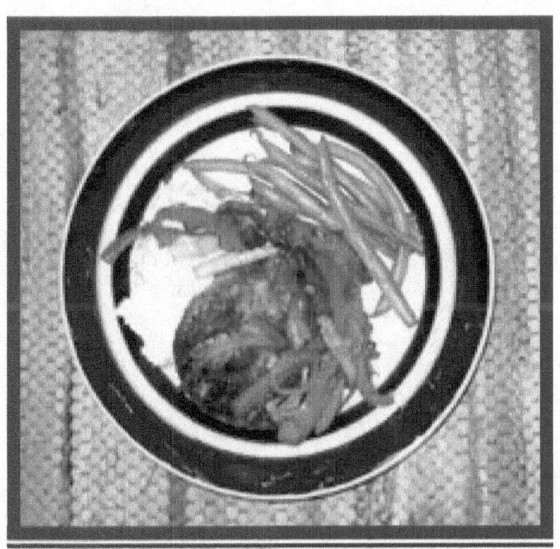

Tip of the Day: **Plan to be on a diet the rest of your life**. Not necessarily a weight reducing diet. At some point you'll want to just maintain your weight. But you will still need to continue to make good healthy food choices – and not slip back to your old eating habits.

Recipe adapted from: ***Weight Maintenance - Metric Edition*** with permission of NoPaperPress.com.

Appendix A Weight Loss Prediction Tables - Men

This appendix contains 36 Weight Loss Prediction Tables for Men. The tables cover men from 18 to 75 years, with heights ranging from 150 to 195 cm, and activity levels from 0 to 4. Refer to the index shown in Table AA below to find the table that's right for you. Before choosing your personal Weight Loss Prediction table, you must determine your Activity Level (see **Table 1** on page 18).

Age	Height	Activity Levels	Table Numbers Page Number
18 - 35	150 to 165 cm	1 to 4	A.1 to A.4 Page 55
18 - 35	166 to 180 cm	1 to 4	A.5 to A.8 Page 59
18 - 35	181 to 195 cm	1 to 4	A.9 to A.12 Page 63
36 - 55	150 to 165 cm	0 to 3	A.13 to A.16 Page 67
36 - 55	166 to 180 cm	0 to 3	A.17 to A.20 Page 71
36 - 55	181 to 195 cm	0 to 3	A.21 to A.24 Page 75
56 - 75	150 to 165 cm	0 to 3	A.25 to A.28 Page 79
56 - 75	166 to 180 cm	0 to 3	A.29 to A.32 Page 83
56 - 75	181 to 195 cm	0 to 3	A.33 to A.36 Page 87

Table AA: 36 Weight Loss Prediction Tables for Men

Once you have selected the Weight Loss Prediction table that's appropriate for you, return to **Example 1** (page 36) for instruction on how to use the data in the table.

WEIGHT LOSS PREDICTION – MEN   18 to 35 yrs.

Weight Loss	Diet kcal	Present Weight (kg)							
		55	60	70	80	90	100	110	120
2 kg	1200	18	16	13	11	10	9	8	7
	1500	26	22	17	14	12	10	9	8
	1800	49	37	25	19	15	13	11	10
	2100		109	45	29	21	17	14	12
4 kg	1200	37	33	27	23	20	18	16	15
	1500	55	46	35	29	25	21	19	17
	1800	107	79	52	39	32	27	23	20
	2100		263	97	60	44	35	29	25
6 kg	1200		50	41	35	31	27	25	23
	1500		72	55	45	38	33	29	26
	1800		125	81	61	49	41	35	31
	2100			156	95	69	54	45	38
10 kg	1200		89	72	61	53	47	42	39
	1500		72	96	78	65	57	50	45
	1800		241	147	107	85	71	61	54
	2100			311	173	122	95	78	66
15 kg	1200			114	95	82	73	66	60
	1500			156	123	102	88	78	70
	1800			248	174	135	111	95	83
	2100				299	199	151	123	104
20 kg	1200			161	133	114	100	90	82
	1500			226	174	143	122	107	92
	1800				254	192	156	132	115
	2100					295	217	173	145
25 kg	1200	Values in table are time in days to lose weight indicated.			175	149	130	116	105
	1500				234	189	159	139	123
	1800				356	259	207	173	149
	2100						294	230	190
30 kg	1200				222	189	162	143	129
	1500				304	240	200	173	153
	1800					340	264	218	186
	2100							295	240

Table A.1 Weight Loss Prediction: Men, 150 to 165 cm, Activity Level 1

WEIGHT LOSS PREDICTION – MEN   18 to 35 yrs.

Weight Loss	Diet kcal	Present Weight (kg)							
		55	60	70	80	90	100	110	120
2 kg	1200	15	13	11	9	8	7	6	6
	1500	20	17	14	11	10	8	7	7
	1800	32	25	18	14	12	10	9	8
	2100	73	47	27	19	15	12	11	9
4 kg	1200	30	27	22	19	17	15	14	12
	1500	42	36	28	23	20	17	16	14
	1800	67	53	38	30	24	21	18	16
	2100	169	102	58	41	31	26	22	19
6 kg	1200		42	35	30	26	23	21	19
	1500		56	44	36	31	27	24	22
	1800		84	59	46	38	32	28	25
	2100		168	91	63	49	40	34	29
10 kg	1200		74	60	51	45	40	36	33
	1500		100	77	62	53	46	41	37
	1800		156	105	80	65	55	48	43
	2100			169	113	85	69	58	50
15 kg	1200			95	80	69	61	55	50
	1500			123	99	83	72	64	57
	1800			174	129	104	87	75	66
	2100			303	187	137	109	91	79
20 kg	1200			134	112	96	85	76	69
	1500			177	140	116	100	88	79
	1800			262	186	146	121	104	91
	2100				282	198	155	128	109
25 kg	1200	Values in table			147	125	110	98	88
	1500	are time in days			186	152	130	114	101
	1800	to lose weight			255	195	159	136	118
	2100	indicated.				273	207	168	142
30 kg	1200				186	157	136	121	109
	1500				240	193	163	141	125
	1800				343	252	202	170	147
	2100					368	268	214	179

Table A.2 Weight Loss Prediction: Men , 150 to 165 cm, Activity Level 2

WEIGHT LOSS PREDICTION – MEN   18 to 35 yrs.

Weight Loss	Diet kcal	Present Weight (kg)							
		55	**60**	**70**	**80**	**90**	**100**	**110**	**120**
2 kg	1200	11	10	9	7	6	6	5	5
	1500	15	13	10	9	7	6	6	5
	1800	20	17	13	10	9	7	6	6
	2100	32	24	17	13	10	9	7	7
4 kg	1200	24	22	18	15	13	12	11	10
	1500	31	27	21	18	15	14	12	11
	1800	43	35	27	21	18	15	14	12
	2100	69	52	35	27	22	18	16	14
6 kg	1200		33	28	24	21	18	17	15
	1500		42	33	28	24	21	19	17
	1800		55	41	33	28	24	21	19
	2100		82	55	41	33	28	24	21
10 kg	1200		58	48	41	36	32	29	26
	1500		74	58	48	41	36	32	29
	1800		100	73	58	48	41	36	32
	2100		156	99	73	58	48	42	36
15 kg	1200			76	64	56	49	44	40
	1500			92	76	64	56	50	45
	1800			119	92	76	64	56	50
	2100			166	118	92	76	65	57
20 kg	1200			107	89	77	68	61	55
	1500			132	106	89	77	68	61
	1800			174	131	106	90	78	69
	2100			256	172	131	107	90	79
25 kg	1200	Values in table are time in days to lose weight indicated.			117	100	88	78	71
	1500				141	117	100	88	79
	1800				177	141	117	101	89
	2100				239	176	141	118	102
30 kg	1200				148	125	109	97	88
	1500				181	148	126	110	98
	1800				232	180	148	126	111
	2100				329	230	180	149	127

Table A.3 Weight Loss Prediction: Men , 150 to 165 cm, Activity Level 3

WEIGHT LOSS PREDICTION – MEN   18 to 35 yrs.

Weight Loss	Diet kcal	Present Weight (kg)							
		55	60	70	80	90	100	110	120
2 kg	1200	8	7	6	5	5	4	4	3
	1500	10	8	7	6	5	4	4	4
	1800	12	10	8	7	6	5	4	4
	2100	15	13	9	8	6	5	5	4
4 kg	1200	17	15	13	11	10	9	8	7
	1500	20	18	15	12	11	9	8	8
	1800	25	21	17	14	12	10	9	8
	2100	32	27	20	16	13	11	10	9
6 kg	1200		24	20	17	15	13	12	11
	1500		28	22	19	16	14	13	12
	1800		33	26	21	18	16	14	13
	2100		42	31	25	21	18	15	14
10 kg	1200		42	34	29	26	23	21	19
	1500		49	39	33	28	25	22	20
	1800		59	46	37	32	28	24	22
	2100		76	55	43	36	31	27	24
15 kg	1200			54	46	40	36	32	29
	1500			63	52	45	39	35	31
	1800			74	59	50	43	38	34
	2100			89	69	57	48	42	37
20 kg	1200			77	64	56	49	44	40
	1500			89	73	62	54	48	43
	1800			106	84	70	60	52	47
	2100			131	99	80	67	58	51
25 kg	1200	Values in table			84	72	64	57	51
	1500	are time in days			96	81	70	62	56
	1800	to lose weight			112	92	78	68	60
	2100	indicated.			133	105	88	75	66
30 kg	1200				107	91	79	70	64
	1500				122	102	87	77	69
	1800				144	116	98	85	75
	2100				175	135	111	94	82

Table A.4 Weight Loss Prediction: Men, 150 to 165 cm, Activity Level 4

WEIGHT LOSS PREDICTION – MEN 18 to 35 yrs.

Weight Loss	Diet kcal	Present Weight (kg)							
		65	**70**	**80**	**90**	**100**	**110**	**120**	**130**
2 kg	1200	13	12	10	9	8	7	7	6
	1500	17	15	13	11	9	8	8	7
	1800	24	21	16	14	12	10	9	8
	2100	44	34	24	18	15	12	11	10
5 kg	1200	34	31	27	23	21	19	17	16
	1500	45	40	33	28	25	22	20	18
	1800	65	56	43	35	30	26	24	21
	2100	122	92	62	48	39	33	28	25
10 kg	1200		65	56	49	44	40	36	33
	1500		85	69	59	52	46	42	38
	1800		122	92	75	63	55	49	44
	2100		215	137	102	82	69	59	52
15 kg	1200			87	76	68	61	56	51
	1500			110	93	80	71	64	59
	1800			148	119	99	86	76	68
	2100			230	165	130	108	92	81
20 kg	1200			121	105	93	84	76	70
	1500			155	129	111	98	88	80
	1800			214	168	139	119	105	93
	2100			352	240	184	151	128	112
25 kg	1200				136	120	108	98	90
	1500				169	145	127	113	103
	1800				224	182	155	135	120
	2100				333	247	199	168	145
30 kg	1200	Values in table are time in days to lose weight indicated.			171	149	133	120	110
	1500				214	181	158	140	127
	1800				290	232	194	168	149
	2100					322	254	211	181
35 kg	1200					181	160	144	132
	1500					222	191	169	152
	1800					288	238	204	180
	2100						317	259	220

Table A.5 Weight Loss Prediction: Men, 166 to 180 cm, Activity Level 1

WEIGHT LOSS PREDICTION – MEN 18 to 35 yrs.

Weight Loss	Diet kcal	Present Weight (kg)							
		65	70	80	90	100	110	120	130
2 kg	1200	11	10	9	8	7	6	6	5
	1500	14	12	10	9	8	7	6	6
	1800	18	16	13	11	9	8	7	6
	2100	28	23	17	13	11	10	8	7
5 kg	1200	29	26	23	20	18	16	15	14
	1500	36	32	27	23	21	18	17	15
	1800	49	42	34	28	24	21	19	17
	2100	75	61	45	35	29	25	22	20
10 kg	1200		55	47	42	37	34	31	28
	1500		69	57	49	43	38	35	32
	1800		92	72	59	51	44	40	36
	2100		136	96	75	62	53	46	41
15 kg	1200			74	65	58	52	47	44
	1500			90	77	67	59	54	49
	1800			115	94	79	69	61	55
	2100			158	120	98	83	72	64
20 kg	1200			103	90	79	71	65	60
	1500			127	107	92	82	73	67
	1800			164	132	110	96	85	76
	2100			233	172	138	115	99	88
25 kg	1200				116	102	92	83	76
	1500				140	120	106	95	86
	1800				174	145	124	109	98
	2100				233	183	151	129	113
30 kg	1200	Values in table are time in days to lose weight indicated.			146	127	113	103	94
	1500				176	150	131	117	106
	1800				224	183	155	136	121
	2100				309	235	191	162	141
35 kg	1200					154	137	123	112
	1500					183	159	141	127
	1800					226	190	164	146
	2100					296	236	198	171

Table A.6 Weight Loss Prediction: Men, 166 to 180 cm, Activity Level 2

WEIGHT LOSS PREDICTION – MEN 18 to 35 yrs.

Weight Loss	Diet kcal	Present Weight (kg)							
		65	70	80	90	100	110	120	130
2 kg	1200	9	8	7	6	5	5	4	4
	1500	10	9	8	7	6	5	5	4
	1800	13	12	9	8	7	6	5	5
	2100	17	15	12	9	8	7	6	5
5 kg	1200	23	21	18	16	14	13	12	11
	1500	28	25	21	18	16	14	13	12
	1800	35	31	25	21	18	16	15	13
	2100	46	40	31	25	21	18	16	15
10 kg	1200		45	38	34	30	27	25	23
	1500		53	45	38	34	30	27	25
	1800		66	53	45	39	34	30	28
	2100		87	66	53	45	39	34	31
15 kg	1200			60	53	47	42	38	35
	1500			70	60	53	47	42	39
	1800			84	70	60	53	47	43
	2100			106	84	70	60	53	48
20 kg	1200			84	73	64	58	53	48
	1500			9	84	73	65	58	53
	1800			120	98	84	73	65	59
	2100			153	119	98	84	73	65
25 kg	1200				94	83	75	68	62
	1500				109	94	83	75	68
	1800				130	109	95	84	75
	2100				159	129	110	95	84
30 kg	1200	Values in table		118	103	92	83	76	
	1500	are time in days		138	118	104	93	84	
	1800	to lose weight		165	137	118	104	93	
	2100	indicated.		206	164	138	119	105	
35 kg	1200					125	111	100	91
	1500					144	125	111	100
	1800					169	145	126	112
	2100					205	169	144	126

Table A.7 Weight Loss Prediction: Men, 166 to 180 cm, Activity Level 3

WEIGHT LOSS PREDICTION – MEN 18 to 35 yrs.

Weight Loss	Diet kcal	Present Weight (kg)							
		65	70	80	90	100	110	120	130
2 kg	1200	6	6	5	4	4	3	3	3
	1500	7	7	6	5	4	4	3	3
	1800	8	7	6	5	5	4	4	3
	2100	10	9	7	6	5	4	4	4
5 kg	1200	17	15	13	12	10	9	9	8
	1500	19	18	15	13	11	10	9	9
	1800	22	20	17	14	13	11	10	9
	2100	27	24	19	16	14	12	11	10
10 kg	1200		33	28	25	22	20	18	17
	1500		37	31	27	24	22	20	18
	1800		43	35	30	26	23	21	19
	2100		51	41	34	29	26	23	21
15 kg	1200			44	39	34	31	28	26
	1500			49	43	37	33	30	28
	1800			56	47	41	36	33	30
	2100			65	53	46	40	35	32
20 kg	1200			62	53	47	43	39	35
	1500			69	59	52	46	42	38
	1800			79	66	57	50	45	41
	2100			92	75	64	55	49	44
25 kg	1200				69	61	55	50	45
	1500				77	67	59	53	49
	1800				87	74	65	58	52
	2100				99	83	72	63	57
30 kg	1200	Values in table are time in days to lose weight indicated.			87	76	68	61	56
	1500				97	84	74	66	60
	1800				110	93	81	72	65
	2100				126	105	90	79	70
35 kg	1200					92	82	74	67
	1500					102	89	80	72
	1800					114	98	87	78
	2100					129	109	95	84

Table A.8 Weight Loss Prediction: Men, 166 to 180 cm, Activity Level 4

WEIGHT LOSS PREDICTION – MEN 18 to 35 yrs.

Weight Loss	Diet kcal	Present Weight (kg)							
		75	80	90	100	110	120	130	140
5 kg	1200	27	25	22	20	18	17	15	14
	1500	33	30	26	23	21	19	17	16
	1800	43	39	32	26	24	22	20	18
	2100	63	54	42	35	30	26	23	21
10 kg	1200		52	46	41	37	34	32	30
	1500		64	55	48	43	39	36	33
	1800		83	68	58	51	45	41	38
	2100		117	90	73	62	54	48	43
15 kg	1200			71	64	58	53	49	45
	1500			86	75	67	60	55	51
	1800			107	91	79	70	64	58
	2100			144	116	98	85	75	67
20 kg	1200			98	87	79	72	67	62
	1500			119	103	92	83	75	69
	1800			151	127	110	97	87	79
	2100			207	164	136	117	103	92
25 kg	1200				113	101	92	85	79
	1500				134	118	106	97	89
	1800				166	143	125	112	102
	2100				218	179	152	133	119
30 kg	1200				140	125	114	104	97
	1500				168	147	131	119	109
	1800				210	178	156	139	125
	2100				281	227	191	166	147
35 kg	1200	Values in table				151	136	125	115
	1500	are time in days				178	158	143	130
	1800	to lose weight				218	189	167	150
	2100	indicated.				281	234	201	177
40 kg	1200					178	160	146	134
	1500					211	187	168	153
	1800					261	224	197	177
	2100					344	282	240	210

Table A.9 Weight Loss Prediction: Men35, 181 to 195 cm, Activity Level 1

WEIGHT LOSS PREDICTION – MEN 18 to 35 yrs.

Weight Loss	Diet kcal	Present Weight (kg)							
		75	80	90	100	110	120	130	140
5 kg	1200	23	21	19	17	15	14	13	12
	1500	27	25	22	19	17	16	15	13
	1800	34	31	26	23	20	18	16	15
	2100	45	40	32	27	23	21	19	17
10 kg	1200		45	39	35	32	29	27	25
	1500		53	46	40	36	33	30	28
	1800		66	55	47	42	37	34	31
	2100		86	68	57	49	43	39	35
15 kg	1200			61	55	50	45	42	39
	1500			72	63	56	51	46	43
	1800			86	74	65	58	52	48
	2100			109	90	77	67	60	54
20 kg	1200			85	75	68	62	57	53
	1500			100	87	77	70	64	59
	1800			121	103	90	80	72	65
	2100			155	126	106	93	82	74
25 kg	1200				97	87	79	73	68
	1500				113	100	90	81	75
	1800				134	116	103	92	84
	2100				166	139	120	106	95
30 kg	1200				120	108	98	90	83
	1500				141	124	111	100	92
	1800				169	145	127	114	103
	2100				212	175	150	132	118
35 kg	1200	Values in table are time in days to lose weight indicated.				130	117	107	99
	1500					149	133	120	110
	1800					176	154	137	124
	2100					216	183	159	142
40 kg	1200					153	138	125	115
	1500					177	157	141	129
	1800					211	183	162	145
	2100					262	219	189	167

Table A.10 Weight Loss Prediction: Men, 181 to 195 cm, Activity Level 2

WEIGHT LOSS PREDICTION – MEN 18 to 35 yrs.

Weight Loss	Diet kcal	Present Weight (kg)							
		75	80	90	100	110	120	130	140
5 kg	1200	19	17	15	14	13	11	11	10
	1500	22	20	17	15	14	13	12	11
	1800	26	23	20	17	15	14	13	12
	2100	32	28	23	20	17	16	14	13
10 kg	1200		37	32	29	26	24	22	21
	1500		42	37	32	29	26	24	22
	1800		50	42	37	32	29	26	24
	2100		61	50	42	37	32	29	27
15 kg	1200			50	45	41	37	34	32
	1500			57	50	45	41	37	34
	1800			66	57	50	45	41	37
	2100			78	66	57	50	45	41
20 kg	1200			69	62	56	51	47	43
	1500			79	69	62	56	51	47
	1800			92	79	69	62	56	51
	2100			111	92	79	70	62	56
25 kg	1200				80	72	65	60	55
	1500				90	80	72	65	60
	1800				103	90	80	72	66
	2100				121	103	90	80	72
30 kg	1200				99	88	80	73	68
	1500				112	99	89	80	74
	1800				129	112	99	89	81
	2100				153	129	112	99	89
35 kg	1200	Values in table are time in days to lose weight indicated.				106	96	88	81
	1500					119	106	96	88
	1800					136	119	107	97
	2100					158	136	120	107
40 kg	1200					126	113	103	94
	1500					142	126	113	103
	1800					162	142	126	114
	2100					190	162	142	127

Table A.11 Weight Loss Prediction: Men, 181 to 195 cm, Activity Level 3

WEIGHT LOSS PREDICTION – MEN 18 to 35 yrs.

Weight Loss	Diet kcal	Present Weight (kg)							
		75	80	90	100	110	120	130	140
5 kg	1200	14	13	11	10	9	8	8	7
	1500	15	14	12	11	10	9	8	8
	1800	17	16	14	12	11	10	9	8
	2100	20	18	15	13	12	10	9	9
10 kg	1200		27	24	21	19	18	16	15
	1500		30	26	23	21	19	17	16
	1800		34	29	25	23	20	19	17
	2100		39	32	28	25	22	20	18
15 kg	1200			37	33	30	27	25	23
	1500			41	36	32	29	27	25
	1800			45	40	35	32	29	26
	2100			51	44	38	34	31	28
20 kg	1200			52	46	41	38	35	32
	1500			57	50	45	40	37	34
	1800			63	55	48	43	39	36
	2100			71	61	53	47	42	39
25 kg	1200				59	53	48	44	41
	1500				65	58	52	47	43
	1800				71	63	56	51	46
	2100				79	69	61	55	50
30 kg	1200				74	66	59	54	50
	1500				81	71	64	58	53
	1800				89	78	69	63	57
	2100				100	86	76	68	61
35 kg	1200	Values in table				79	71	65	60
	1500	are time in days				86	77	70	64
	1800	to lose weight				94	84	75	68
	2100	indicated.				105	91	81	73
40 kg	1200					93	84	76	70
	1500					102	91	82	75
	1800					112	99	88	80
	2100					125	109	96	86

Table A.12 Weight Loss Prediction: Men, 181 to 195 cm, Activity Level 4

WEIGHT LOSS PREDICTION – MEN 36 to 55 yrs.

Weight Loss	Diet kcal	Present Weight (kg)							
		55	60	70	80	90	100	110	120
2 kg	1200	22	19	16	13	11	10	9	8
	1500	36	29	22	17	15	13	11	10
	1800	100	62	36	26	20	16	14	12
	2100			101	48	31	24	19	16
4 kg	1200	45	40	32	27	24	21	19	17
	1500	76	62	45	36	30	26	23	21
	1800	234	136	76	53	41	34	29	25
	2100			233	102	66	49	39	33
6 kg	1200		61	49	42	36	32	29	26
	1500		96	70	55	46	40	35	31
	1800		226	120	83	64	52	44	39
	2100				162	102	76	60	50
10 kg	1200		108	86	72	62	55	50	45
	1500		177	124	97	80	69	60	54
	1800			223	148	112	91	77	66
	2100				315	186	134	105	87
15 kg	1200			137	113	97	85	77	69
	1500			203	155	126	107	93	83
	1800				246	180	144	120	103
	2100					317	218	168	137
20 kg	1200			195	159	135	118	105	95
	1500			301	222	178	149	129	114
	1800					260	203	168	143
	2100						320	239	193
25 kg	1200	Values in table are time in days to lose weight indicated.			210	176	153	136	122
	1500				301	236	195	168	148
	1800						271	221	187
	2100							323	255
30 kg	1200				268	222	191	168	151
	1500					302	247	210	183
	1800							280	235
	2100								327

Table A.13 Weight Loss Prediction: Men, 150 to 165 cm, Activity Level 0

WEIGHT LOSS PREDICTION – MEN 36 to 55 yrs.

Weight Loss	Diet kcal	Present Weight (kg)							
		55	60	70	80	90	100	110	120
2 kg	1200	20	17	14	12	10	9	8	8
	1500	30	25	19	15	13	11	10	9
	1800	67	46	29	21	17	14	12	11
	2100		272	61	35	25	19	16	13
4 kg	1200	41	36	29	25	22	19	17	16
	1500	64	53	40	32	27	23	20	18
	1800	148	100	61	45	35	29	25	22
	2100			134	74	52	40	33	28
6 kg	1200		55	45	38	33	29	26	24
	1500		83	61	49	41	35	31	28
	1800		162	96	69	54	45	39	34
	2100			223	117	80	62	50	42
10 kg	1200		98	78	66	57	50	45	41
	1500		150	108	86	71	61	54	48
	1800		327	176	123	95	78	67	58
	2100				219	144	108	87	73
15 kg	1200			124	103	89	78	70	63
	1500			176	136	112	96	84	75
	1800			306	202	152	123	104	91
	2100					240	175	138	115
20 kg	1200			176	144	123	107	96	87
	1500			259	194	167	133	116	102
	1800				299	219	174	145	125
	2100						253	196	161
25 kg	1200	Values in table			190	160	139	124	111
	1500	are time in days			262	208	174	150	132
	1800	to lose weight				297	231	191	163
	2100	indicated.					349	262	212
30 kg	1200					242	202	174	153	137
	1500						266	219	187	164
	1800							297	241	204
	2100								341	270

Table A.14 Weight Loss Prediction: Men, 150 to 165 cm, Activity Level 1

WEIGHT LOSS PREDICTION – MEN 36 to 55 yrs.

Weight Loss	Diet kcal	Present Weight (kg)							
		55	60	70	80	90	100	110	120
2 kg	1200	16	14	12	10	9	8	7	6
	1500	23	19	15	12	10	9	8	7
	1800	38	30	20	16	13	11	9	8
	2100	120	63	33	22	17	14	11	10
4 kg	1200	33	29	24	20	18	16	14	13
	1500	47	40	31	25	21	19	17	15
	1800	82	62	43	33	27	22	20	17
	2100	310	141	69	46	35	28	24	21
6 kg	1200		45	37	31	27	24	22	20
	1500		62	48	39	33	29	25	23
	1800		99	67	51	41	35	30	26
	2100		242	110	72	54	44	37	31
10 kg	1200		80	65	54	47	42	38	34
	1500		112	84	68	57	49	44	39
	1800		187	120	89	71	60	52	46
	2100			210	130	96	76	63	54
15 kg	1200			102	86	74	65	58	53
	1500			135	107	89	77	68	61
	1800			200	144	113	94	81	71
	2100				220	155	121	100	85
20 kg	1200			145	120	102	90	80	72
	1500			196	152	125	107	93	83
	1800			307	209	161	132	112	98
	2100				341	227	172	140	118
25 kg	1200	Values in table			157	133	116	103	93
	1500	are time in days			204	165	139	121	107
	1800	to lose weight			290	216	174	146	127
	2100	indicated.				316	232	185	155
30 kg	1200					201	167	145	128	115
	1500					265	209	175	151	133
	1800						281	221	184	158
	2100						303	236	195

Table A.15 Weight Loss Prediction: Men, 150 to 165 cm, Activity Level 2

WEIGHT LOSS PREDICTION – MEN 36 to 55 yrs.

Weight Loss	Diet kcal	Present Weight (kg)							
		55	60	70	80	90	100	110	120
2. kg	1200	12	11	9	8	7	6	5	5
	1500	16	14	11	9	8	7	6	5
	1800	23	19	14	11	9	8	7	6
	2100	38	28	19	14	11	9	8	7
4 kg	1200	26	23	19	16	14	13	11	10
	1500	33	29	23	19	16	14	13	11
	1800	48	39	29	23	19	16	14	13
	2100	84	60	39	29	23	19	17	15
6 kg	1200		35	29	25	22	19	17	16
	1500		45	35	29	25	22	19	18
	1800		61	45	35	29	25	22	20
	2100		97	61	45	36	30	25	22
10 kg	1200		62	51	43	37	33	30	27
	1500		80	62	51	43	38	33	30
	1800		112	80	62	51	44	38	34
	2100		188	111	80	63	52	44	39
15 kg	1200			80	67	58	52	46	42
	1500			99	80	68	59	52	47
	1800			130	99	81	68	59	53
	2100			190	130	100	82	69	60
20 kg	1200			113	94	81	71	64	58
	1500			142	113	95	81	72	64
	1800			192	142	114	95	82	72
	2100			300	191	143	115	96	83
25 kg	1200	Values in table			124	105	92	82	74
	1500	are time in days			151	124	106	93	83
	1800	to lose weight			193	151	125	107	94
	2100	indicated.			270	193	152	126	108
30 kg	1200				157	132	115	101	91
	1500				194	157	133	115	102
	1800				255	194	158	134	117
	2100					255	195	159	135

Table A.16 Weight Loss Prediction: Men, 150 to 165 cm, Activity Level 3

WEIGHT LOSS PREDICTION – MEN   36 to 55 yrs.

Weight Loss	Diet kcal	Present Weight (kg)							
		65	70	80	90	100	110	120	130
2 kg	1200	16	14	12	11	10	9	8	7
	1500	23	20	16	14	12	10	9	8
	1800	38	31	23	18	15	13	11	10
	2100	118	70	39	27	21	17	14	13
5 kg	1200	42	38	32	28	25	23	21	19
	1500	60	52	42	35	31	27	24	22
	1800	103	83	60	47	39	34	30	27
	2100		203	105	72	55	45	38	33
10 kg	1200		80	68	59	52	47	43	40
	1500		112	89	74	64	57	51	46
	1800		187	130	101	83	71	62	55
	2100			243	157	118	95	79	69
15 kg	1200			106	92	81	73	66	61
	1500			142	117	100	88	78	71
	1800			214	162	131	111	96	85
	2100				263	190	150	125	107
20 kg	1200			148	127	111	100	90	83
	1500			202	164	139	121	108	97
	1800			318	232	185	154	133	117
	2100					276	213	174	148
25 kg	1200				165	144	128	116	106
	1500				217	181	157	139	125
	1800				315	245	202	173	152
	2100						285	230	194
30 kg	1200	Values in table		208	180	159	143	130
	1500	are time in days		277	229	196	172	154
	1800	to lose weight			315	256	217	189
	2100	indicated.					293	243
35 kg	1200					218	192	172	156
	1500					281	239	208	185
	1800						316	265	229
	2100								298

Table A.17 Weight Loss Prediction: Men, 166 to 180 cm, Activity Level 0

WEIGHT LOSS PREDICTION – MEN 36 to 55 yrs

Weight Loss	Diet kcal	Present Weight (kg)							
		65	70	80	90	100	110	120	130
2 kg	1200	14	13	11	10	9	8	7	7
	1500	20	17	14	12	11	9	8	8
	1800	31	26	19	16	13	11	10	9
	2100	70	48	30	22	17	14	12	11
5 kg	1200	38	35	29	26	23	21	19	17
	1500	52	46	37	32	26	24	22	20
	1800	83	69	51	41	34	30	26	24
	2100	206	135	81	58	46	38	32	28
10 kg	1200		73	62	54	48	43	39	36
	1500		99	79	67	58	51	46	42
	1800		153	110	87	72	62	55	49
	2100		341	182	126	98	80	68	59
15 kg	1200			97	84	74	67	61	56
	1500			126	105	90	79	71	64
	1800			180	139	114	97	85	76
	2100			317	208	156	126	106	92
20 kg	1200			136	116	102	91	83	76
	1500			179	146	125	109	97	88
	1800			264	198	160	135	117	104
	2100				309	224	178	148	128
25 kg	1200				151	132	118	106	97
	1500				193	163	141	125	113
	1800				267	212	177	152	134
	2100					306	237	195	166
30 kg	1200	Values in table			190	164	146	131	119
	1500	are time in days			246	204	176	155	139
	1800	to lose weight			351	271	223	190	167
	2100	indicated.					305	246	208
35 kg	1200					200	176	157	143
	1500					251	214	187	167
	1800					340	275	232	202
	2100							305	254

Table A.18 Weight Loss Prediction: Men, 166 to 180 cm, Activity Level 1

WEIGHT LOSS PREDICTION – MEN 36 to 55 yrs

Weight Loss	Diet kcal	Present Weight (kg)							
		65	70	80	90	100	110	120	130
2 kg	1200	12	11	9	8	7	7	6	5
	1500	16	14	11	10	9	8	7	6
	1800	22	19	15	12	10	9	8	7
	2100	36	28	20	15	13	11	9	8
5 kg	1200	32	29	25	22	19	17	16	15
	1500	41	37	30	26	22	20	18	16
	1800	58	50	38	32	27	23	21	19
	2100	100	77	53	41	33	28	25	22
10 kg	1200		61	52	45	40	36	33	30
	1500		78	64	54	47	42	37	34
	1800		108	82	67	56	49	43	39
	2100		177	116	88	71	59	51	45
15 kg	1200			81	70	62	56	51	47
	1500			101	85	73	65	58	53
	1800			132	106	88	76	67	60
	2100			194	141	112	93	80	70
20 kg	1200			114	98	86	77	70	64
	1500			142	118	101	89	80	72
	1800			191	150	124	106	93	83
	2100			294	205	159	130	111	97
25 kg	1200				127	111	99	90	82
	1500				155	132	115	103	93
	1800				200	163	138	120	107
	2100				282	212	172	145	126
30 kg	1200	Values in table		159	138	123	110	101
	1500	are time in days		197	166	143	127	114
	1800	to lose weight		259	206	173	150	132
	2100	indicated.			276	218	182	157
35 kg	1200					168	148	133	120
	1500					203	174	153	137
	1800					257	212	182	160
	2100						273	224	191

Table A.19 Weight Loss Prediction: Men, 166 to 180 cm, Activity Level 2

WEIGHT LOSS PREDICTION – MEN 36 to 55 yrs

Weight Loss	Diet kcal	Present Weight (kg)							
		65	70	80	90	100	110	120	130
2 kg	1200	9	9	7	6	6	5	5	4
	1500	12	10	9	7	7	6	5	5
	1800	15	13	10	9	7	7	6	5
	2100	20	17	13	10	9	8	7	6
5 kg	1200	25	23	20	17	15	14	13	12
	1500	31	28	23	20	17	15	14	13
	1800	39	34	28	23	20	17	16	14
	2100	55	46	34	28	23	20	18	16
10 kg	1200		49	41	36	32	29	26	24
	1500		59	49	41	36	32	29	27
	1800		74	59	49	42	37	33	29
	2100		101	74	59	49	42	37	33
15 kg	1200			65	56	50	45	41	37
	1500			77	65	57	50	45	41
	1800			94	77	65	57	51	46
	2100			121	94	77	66	58	51
20 kg	1200			90	78	69	62	56	51
	1500			108	91	78	69	62	56
	1800			134	108	91	79	70	63
	2100			176	134	109	92	80	70
25 kg	1200				101	89	79	72	66
	1500				119	102	89	80	72
	1800				143	119	102	90	81
	2100				180	144	120	103	91
30 kg	1200	Values in table		127	111	98	88	81
	1500	are time in days		150	127	111	99	89
	1800	to lose weight		183	150	128	112	100
	2100	indicated.		236	183	151	129	113
35 kg	1200					134	118	106	96
	1500					155	135	119	107
	1800					185	156	136	120
	2100					230	186	157	137

Table A.20 Weight Loss Prediction: Men, 166 to 180 cm, Activity Level 3

WEIGHT LOSS PREDICTION – MEN 36 to 55 yrs

Weight Loss	Diet kcal	Present Weight (kg)							
		75	80	90	100	110	120	130	140
5 kg	1200	31	29	25	23	21	19	18	16
	1500	40	36	31	27	24	22	20	19
	1800	56	49	40	34	30	26	24	22
	2100	93	76	56	45	38	32	29	26
10 kg	1200		60	53	47	43	39	36	34
	1500		77	65	57	51	46	42	38
	1800		106	85	71	62	55	49	45
	2100		169	122	96	79	68	59	53
15 kg	1200			82	73	66	60	56	52
	1500			102	89	78	71	64	59
	1800			135	112	96	85	76	69
	2100			198	152	125	106	92	82
20 kg	1200			114	101	91	83	76	71
	1500			143	123	108	97	88	81
	1800			191	157	134	117	104	94
	2100			292	218	175	147	128	113
25 kg	1200				130	117	106	97	90
	1500				160	140	125	113	103
	1800				207	174	151	134	121
	2100				294	232	193	166	146
30 kg	1200				162	144	130	119	110
	1500				200	174	154	139	127
	1800				263	219	189	166	149
	2100					297	244	207	181
35 kg	1200	Values in table				173	156	143	132
	1500	are time in days				211	186	167	152
	1800	to lose weight				269	229	201	179
	2100	indicated.					300	253	220
40 kg	1200					205	184	167	154
	1500					251	220	196	178
	1800					325	274	238	212
	2100							304	261

Table A.21 Weight Loss Prediction: Men, 181 to 195 cm, Activity Level 0

WEIGHT LOSS PREDICTION – MEN 36 to 55 yrs

Weight Loss	Diet kcal	Present Weight (kg)							
		75	80	90	100	110	120	130	140
5 kg	1200	29	27	23	21	19	17	16	15
	1500	36	33	28	25	22	20	18	17
	1800	49	43	35	30	26	24	21	19
	2100	74	62	48	39	33	28	25	23
10 kg	1200		56	49	44	40	36	33	31
	1500		69	59	52	46	42	38	35
	1800		92	75	63	55	49	44	40
	2100		137	102	82	69	59	52	47
15 kg	1200			76	68	61	56	51	48
	1500			93	80	71	64	59	54
	1800			119	99	86	76	68	62
	2100			165	130	108	92	81	72
20 kg	1200			105	93	84	76	70	65
	1500			129	111	98	88	80	74
	1800			168	139	119	105	93	85
	2100			240	184	151	128	112	100
25 kg	1200				120	108	98	90	83
	1500				145	127	113	103	94
	1800				182	155	135	120	109
	2100				247	199	168	145	128
30 kg	1200				149	133	120	110	102
	1500				181	158	140	127	116
	1800				232	194	168	149	134
	2100					254	211	181	159
35 kg	1200	Values in table			181	160	144	132	121
	1500	are time in days			222	191	169	152	138
	1800	to lose weight			288	238	204	180	161
	2100	indicated.				317	259	220	193
40 kg	1200				215	189	170	154	142
	1500				267	228	200	179	162
	1800					287	244	213	190
	2100						313	263	228

Table A.22 Weight Loss Prediction: Men, 181 to 195 cm, Activity Level 1

WEIGHT LOSS PREDICTION – MEN 36 to 55 yrs

Weight Loss	Diet kcal	Present Weight (kg)							
		75	80	90	100	110	120	130	140
5 kg	1200	24	23	20	18	16	15	14	13
	1500	30	27	23	21	18	17	15	14
	1800	38	34	28	24	21	19	17	16
	2100	51	45	35	29	25	22	20	18
10 kg	1200		47	42	37	34	31	28	26
	1500		57	49	43	38	35	32	29
	1800		72	59	51	44	40	36	33
	2100		96	75	62	53	46	41	37
15 kg	1200			65	58	52	47	44	41
	1500			77	67	59	54	49	45
	1800			94	79	69	61	55	50
	2100			120	98	83	72	64	57
20 kg	1200			90	79	71	65	60	55
	1500			107	92	82	73	67	61
	1800			132	110	96	85	76	69
	2100			172	138	115	99	88	79
25 kg	1200				102	92	83	76	71
	1500				120	106	95	86	79
	1800				145	124	109	98	89
	2100				183	151	129	113	101
30 kg	1200				127	113	103	94	87
	1500				150	131	117	106	97
	1800				183	155	136	121	109
	2100				235	191	162	141	125
35 kg	1200	Values in table are time in days to lose weight indicated.				137	123	112	103
	1500					159	141	127	116
	1800					190	164	146	131
	2100					236	198	171	151
40 kg	1200					161	145	132	121
	1500					189	166	149	135
	1800					228	196	172	154
	2100					289	238	204	179

Table A.23 Weight Loss Prediction: Men, 181 to 195 cm, Activity Level 2

WEIGHT LOSS PREDICTION – MEN 36 to 55 yrs

Weight Loss	Diet kcal	Present Weight (kg)							
		75	80	90	100	110	120	130	140
5 kg	1200	20	18	20	14	13	12	11	10
	1500	23	21	23	16	14	13	12	11
	1800	28	25	28	18	16	15	13	12
	2100	34	31	35	21	18	16	15	13
10 kg	1200		38	34	30	27	25	23	21
	1500		45	38	34	30	27	25	23
	1800		53	45	39	34	30	28	25
	2100		66	53	45	39	34	31	28
15 kg	1200			53	47	42	38	35	33
	1500			60	53	47	42	39	36
	1800			70	60	53	47	43	39
	2100			84	70	60	53	48	43
20 kg	1200			73	64	58	53	48	45
	1500			84	73	65	58	53	49
	1800			98	84	73	65	59	53
	2100			119	98	84	73	65	59
25 kg	1200				83	75	68	62	57
	1500				94	83	75	68	62
	1800				109	95	84	75	68
	2100				129	110	95	84	76
30 kg	1200				103	92	83	76	70
	1500				137	104	93	84	77
	1800				164	118	104	93	84
	2100					138	119	105	94
35 kg	1200	Values in table				111	100	91	84
	1500	are time in days				125	111	100	92
	1800	to lose weight				144	126	112	101
	2100	indicated.				169	144	126	113
40 kg	1200					131	118	107	98
	1500					149	131	118	107
	1800					172	149	132	119
	2100					204	172	150	133

Table A.24 Weight Loss Prediction: Men, 181 to 195 cm, Activity Level 3

WEIGHT LOSS PREDICTION – MEN 56 to 75 yrs

Weight Loss	Diet kcal	Present Weight (kg)							
		55	60	70	80	90	100	110	120
2 kg	1200	25	22	17	15	13	11	10	9
	1500	45	36	25	20	16	14	12	11
	1800	238	100	47	31	23	19	16	14
	2100			289	70	41	29	22	18
4 kg	1200	52	45	36	30	26	23	20	19
	1500	97	75	53	41	34	29	25	22
	1800		229	100	65	49	39	33	28
	2100				154	85	60	46	38
6 kg	1200		70	55	46	40	35	31	28
	1500		119	82	63	52	44	39	34
	1800			160	101	75	60	50	43
	2100				254	135	93	71	58
10 kg	1200		124	97	80	68	60	54	49
	1500		222	147	111	90	76	66	59
	1800			311	184	133	105	87	74
	2100					251	166	125	101
15 kg	1200			154	126	107	93	83	75
	1500			244	179	143	119	103	91
	1800				314	216	167	136	116
	2100						276	202	160
20 kg	1200			221	177	149	129	114	103
	1500				259	202	168	143	125
	1800					317	238	192	161
	2100							292	226
25 kg	1200	Values in table			235	195	167	147	132
	1500	are time in days				270	220	186	162
	1800	to lose weight					321	254	211
	2100	indicated.							303
30 kg	1200				301	246	209	183	163
	1500					279		234	202
	1800							325	266
	2100								

Table A.25 Weight Loss Prediction: Men, 150 to 165 cm, Activity Level 0

WEIGHT LOSS PREDICTION – MEN 56 to 75 yrs

Weight Loss	Diet kcal	Present Weight (kg)							
		55	60	70	80	90	100	110	120
2 kg	1200	22	19	16	13	11	10	9	8
	1500	37	30	22	17	14	12	11	10
	1800	108	64	36	25	20	16	14	12
	2100			101	46	30	23	18	15
4 kg	1200	46	40	32	27	23	21	19	17
	1500	78	63	45	36	30	25	22	20
	1800	259	142	76	53	40	33	28	24
	2100			236	99	63	47	37	31
6 kg	1200		62	50	41	36	32	28	26
	1500		98	70	55	46	39	34	30
	1800		238	120	82	62	51	43	37
	2100				158	99	73	58	48
10 kg	1200		110	87	72	62	54	49	44
	1500		181	125	96	79	67	59	52
	1800			226	147	110	88	74	64
	2100				310	180	129	101	83
15 kg	1200			138	113	96	84	75	68
	1500			206	155	125	105	91	81
	1800			245	177	140	116	100	
	2100					308	210	161	131
20 kg	1200			197	159	134	116	103	93
	1500			307	222	176	147	126	111
	1800					257	199	163	139
	2100						309	230	184
25 kg	1200	Values in table		210	175	151	133	120	
	1500	are time in days		303	234	193	164	144	
	1800	to lose weight				266	215	181	
	2100	indicated.					311	244	
30 kg	1200				270	221	189	165	148
	1500					302	244	206	179
	1800							273	228
	2100								314

Table A.26 Weight Loss Prediction: Men, 150 to 165 cm, Activity Level 1

WEIGHT LOSS PREDICTION – MEN 56 to 75 yrs

Weight Loss	Diet kcal	Present Weight (kg)							
		55	60	70	80	90	100	110	120
2 kg	1200	18	16	13	11	9	8	7	7
	1500	26	22	16	13	11	10	9	8
	1800	49	36	24	18	14	12	10	9
	2100		101	41	26	19	15	13	11
4 kg	1200	37	32	26	22	19	17	15	14
	1500	55	46	34	28	23	20	18	16
	1800	107	77	49	37	29	25	21	19
	2100		244	89	55	40	32	26	22
6 kg	1200		50	40	34	29	26	23	21
	1500		71	53	43	36	31	27	24
	1800		123	77	57	45	38	32	29
	2100			143	86	62	49	40	34
10 kg	1200		88	70	59	51	45	40	36
	1500		129	94	74	62	53	47	42
	1800		240	141	101	79	66	56	49
	2100			286	158	110	86	70	60
15 kg	1200			112	92	79	69	62	56
	1500			152	118	97	83	73	65
	1800			240	165	127	103	88	76
	2100				273	181	137	111	93
20 kg	1200			159	129	110	96	85	77
	1500			223	168	137	116	100	89
	1800				242	181	145	122	106
	2100					269	197	156	130
25 kg	1200		Values in table are time in days to lose weight indicated.		171	144	124	110	99
	1500				227	181	151	130	115
	1800				342	245	193	160	137
	2100						267	208	171
30 kg	1200				218	181	155	136	122
	1500				298	231	190	163	143
	1800					322	247	202	172
	2100						355	267	216

Table A.27 Weight Loss Prediction: Men, 150 to 165 cm, Activity Level 2

WEIGHT LOSS PREDICTION – MEN 56 to 75 yrs

Weight Loss	Diet kcal	Present Weight (kg)							
		55	60	70	80	90	100	110	120
2 kg	1200	13	12	10	8	7	6	6	5
	1500	18	15	12	10	8	7	6	6
	1800	26	21	15	12	10	8	7	6
	2100	49	34	21	15	12	10	9	7
4 kg	1200	28	25	20	17	15	13	12	11
	1500	37	32	25	20	17	15	13	12
	1800	56	44	32	25	21	18	15	14
	2100	110	74	45	32	25	21	18	16
6 kg	1200		38	31	26	23	20	18	17
	1500		49	38	31	27	23	21	18
	1800		70	49	39	32	27	23	21
	2100		120	70	50	39	32	27	24
10 kg	1200		67	54	46	40	35	31	28
	1500		88	67	55	46	40	35	32
	1800		129	88	68	55	47	40	36
	2100		243	129	89	69	56	47	41
15 kg	1200			86	72	62	54	49	44
	1500			108	86	72	62	55	49
	1800			146	109	87	73	63	56
	2100			225	147	110	89	74	64
20 kg	1200			122	100	86	75	67	60
	1500			156	122	101	86	76	68
	1800			218	157	123	102	89	77
	2100				219	158	125	104	89
25 kg	1200	Values in table		132	112	97	86	77
	1500	are time in days		163	133	113	98	87
	1800	to lose weight		214	164	134	114	99
	2100	indicated.		315	216	167	136	116
30 kg	1200				168	140	121	107	96
	1500				211	169	141	122	108
	1800				286	212	170	143	124
	2100					288	215	173	145

Table A.28 Weight Loss Prediction: Men, 150 to 165 cm, Activity Level 3

WEIGHT LOSS PREDICTION – MEN 56 to 75 yrs

Weight Loss	Diet kcal	Present Weight (kg)							
		65	70	80	90	100	110	120	130
2 kg	1200	18	16	14	12	10	9	9	8
	1500	26	23	18	15	13	11	10	9
	1800	51	39	27	21	17	15	13	11
	2100		131	54	34	25	20	17	14
5 kg	1200	47	42	36	31	27	25	22	21
	1500	70	61	48	40	34	30	27	24
	1800	140	106	72	55	45	38	33	29
	2100			149	91	66	52	43	37
10 kg	1200		90	75	64	57	51	46	42
	1500		131	102	83	71	62	55	50
	1800		247	159	118	95	80	69	61
	2100				204	143	111	91	78
15 kg	1200			117	100	88	79	71	65
	1500			163	132	111	97	86	77
	1800			266	191	151	125	107	94
	2100					235	178	144	122
20 kg	1200			165	139	122	108	98	89
	1500			233	185	155	134	118	106
	1800				278	214	175	149	130
	2100					348	255	203	170
25 kg	1200				182	158	139	125	114
	1500				246	203	174	152	136
	1800					287	231	195	169
	2100						347	270	222
30 kg	1200	Values in table are time in days to lose weight indicated.			230	197	173	155	140
	1500				317	257	218	190	169
	1800						294	245	211
	2100							345	281
35 kg	1200					239	209	186	168
	1500					318	266	230	203
	1800							301	256
	2100								

Table A.29 Weight Loss Prediction: Men, 166 to 180 cm, Activity Level 0

WEIGHT LOSS PREDICTION – MEN 56 to 75 yrs.

Weight Loss	Diet kcal	Present Weight (kg)							
		65	70	80	90	100	110	120	130
2 kg	1200	16	15	12	11	9	8	8	7
	1500	23	20	16	13	12	10	9	8
	1800	39	31	23	18	15	13	11	10
	2100	127	71	38	27	20	17	14	12
5 kg	1200	42	38	32	28	25	22	20	19
	1500	60	53	42	35	30	27	24	22
	1800	106	84	60	47	39	33	29	26
	2100		209	104	70	53	43	36	32
10 kg	1200		81	68	58	52	46	42	39
	1500		114	89	74	63	55	49	45
	1800		191	130	100	81	69	60	53
	2100			244	155	115	92	76	66
15 kg	1200			106	91	80	72	65	59
	1500			142	116	99	86	77	69
	1800			215	160	129	108	94	83
	2100				260	186	145	120	103
20 kg	1200			149	127	110	98	89	81
	1500			203	163	137	119	105	95
	1800			321	231	182	151	130	114
	2100					270	207	169	143
25 kg	1200				165	143	127	114	104
	1500				216	180	155	136	122
	1800				315	242	198	169	147
	2100						278	222	187
30 kg	1200	Values in table are time in days to lose weight indicated.			208	179	157	141	128
	1500				277	227	193	169	151
	1800					313	251	212	184
	2100							284	235
35 kg	1200					217	190	169	153
	1500					280	236	205	181
	1800						312	259	223
	2100								289

Table A.30 Weight Loss Prediction: Men, 166 to 180 cm, Activity Level 1

WEIGHT LOSS PREDICTION – MEN 56 to 75 yrs

Weight Loss	Diet kcal	Present Weight (kg)							
		65	70	80	90	100	110	120	130
2 kg	1200	13	12	10	9	8	7	6	6
	1500	17	125	13	11	9	8	7	7
	1800	25	21	16	13	11	10	9	8
	2100	47	35	23	18	14	12	10	9
5 kg	1200	35	31	27	23	21	18	17	15
	1500	46	41	33	28	24	21	19	17
	1800	69	57	43	35	29	25	22	20
	2100	134	96	63	47	37	31	27	24
10 kg	1200		66	56	48	43	38	35	32
	1500		87	70	59	51	45	40	36
	1800		126	93	74	62	53	47	42
	2100		231	139	100	79	66	56	49
15 kg	1200			88	76	66	60	54	49
	1500			111	92	79	69	62	56
	1800			151	118	97	83	73	65
	2100			236	163	126	103	88	76
20 kg	1200			123	105	92	82	74	68
	1500			157	129	110	96	85	77
	1800			220	167	136	115	100	89
	2100				240	180	145	122	106
25 kg	1200				137	119	105	95	87
	1500				170	143	124	110	99
	1800				225	180	151	130	115
	2100				337	243	192	160	137
30 kg	1200				172	148	131	117	107
	1500	Values in table are time in days to lose weight indicated.		216	180	155	136	122
	1800				294	230	190	163	143
	2100					319	246	202	172
35 kg	1200					180	158	141	128
	1500					221	188	165	147
	1800					287	234	198	172
	2100						309	249	209

Table A.31 Weight Loss Prediction: Men, 166 to 180 cm, Activity Level 2

WEIGHT LOSS PREDICTION – MEN 56 to 75 yrs

Weight Loss	Diet kcal	Present Weight (kg)							
		65	70	80	90	100	110	120	130
2 kg	1200	10	9	8	7	6	5	5	5
	1500	13	11	9	8	7	6	5	5
	1800	16	14	11	9	8	7	6	6
	2100	24	19	14	11	9	8	7	6
5 kg	1200	27	24	21	18	16	15	13	12
	1500	33	30	25	21	18	16	15	13
	1800	44	38	30	25	21	19	17	15
	2100	64	52	38	30	25	22	19	17
10 kg	1200		52	44	38	34	30	28	25
	1500		64	52	44	38	34	31	28
	1800		82	64	52	45	39	35	31
	2100		117	83	65	53	45	39	35
15 kg	1200			69	59	52	47	43	39
	1500			82	69	60	53	48	43
	1800			102	83	70	61	54	48
	2100			136	103	84	71	61	54
20 kg	1200			96	82	72	65	58	53
	1500			116	97	83	73	65	59
	1800			147	117	98	84	74	66
	2100			200	148	118	99	85	75
25 kg	1200				107	94	83	75	69
	1500				127	108	95	84	76
	1800				155	128	109	96	85
	2100				201	157	130	111	97
30 kg	1200	Values in table			135	117	103	93	84
	1500	are time in days			161	136	118	104	94
	1800	to lose weight			200	162	137	119	105
	2100	indicated.			265	202	164	139	121
35 kg	1200					142	125	111	101
	1500					166	143	126	113
	1800					201	167	144	127
	2100					254	203	170	146

Table A.32 Weight Loss Prediction: Men, 166 to 180 cm, Activity Level 3

WEIGHT LOSS PREDICTION – MEN 56 to 75 yrs

Weight Loss	Diet kcal	Present Weight (kg)							
		75	80	90	100	110	120	130	140
5 kg	1200	34	32	28	25	22	20	19	18
	1500	45	41	35	30	27	24	22	20
	1800	67	58	46	38	33	29	26	24
	2100	128	99	69	53	43	37	32	28
10 kg	1200		66	58	51	46	42	39	36
	1500		87	73	63	55	50	45	42
	1800		126	98	81	69	61	54	49
	2100		227	150	113	92	77	67	59
15 kg	1200			90	80	71	65	60	56
	1500			114	98	86	77	70	64
	1800			157	127	108	94	84	75
	2100			250	183	145	121	104	92
20 kg	1200			125	110	98	89	82	76
	1500			160	136	119	106	96	87
	1800			224	179	151	130	115	103
	2100				264	206	169	145	127
25 kg	1200				142	126	114	105	97
	1500				178	154	136	123	112
	1800				238	197	169	149	133
	2100					275	223	189	164
30 kg	1200				176	156	141	129	118
	1500				223	192	169	152	138
	1800				306	249	212	185	164
	2100						283	237	204
35 kg	1200	Values in table				189	169	154	141
	1500	are time in days				234	204	182	165
	1800	to lose weight				308	258	224	198
	2100	indicated.						290	248
40 kg	1200					223	199	180	165
	1500					279	242	215	194
	1800						310	266	234
	2100							351	296

Table A.33 Weight Loss Prediction: Men, 181 to 195 cm, Activity Level 0

WEIGHT LOSS PREDICTION – MEN 56 to 75 yrs

Weight Loss	Diet kcal	Present Weight (kg)							
		75	80	90	100	110	120	130	140
5 kg	1200	31	29	25	23	20	19	17	16
	1500	40	37	31	27	24	22	20	18
	1800	57	50	40	34	29	26	23	21
	2100	95	77	56	44	37	32	28	25
10 kg	1200		61	53	47	42	39	36	33
	1500		78	65	57	50	45	41	38
	1800		107	85	71	61	54	48	43
	2100		173	122	95	78	66	58	52
15 kg	1200			82	73	66	60	55	51
	1500			102	88	78	70	63	58
	1800			135	111	95	83	74	67
	2100			199	151	123	104	90	80
20 kg	1200			114	100	90	82	75	69
	1500			143	122	107	96	86	79
	1800			192	156	132	115	102	92
	2100			295	217	173	145	125	110
25 kg	1200				130	116	105	96	89
	1500				159	139	123	111	101
	1800				207	173	149	132	118
	2100				294	230	190	162	142
30 kg	1200				162	143	129	118	109
	1500				200	173	153	137	125
	1800				264	218	186	164	146
	2100					295	240	203	177
35 kg	1200	Values in table				173	155	141	130
	1500	are time in days				210	184	165	149
	1800	to lose weight				268	227	198	176
	2100	indicated.					297	248	214
40 kg	1200					205	183	165	152
	1500					251	218	194	175
	1800					325	272	235	208
	2100						298	255	

Table A.34 Weight Loss Prediction: Men, 181 to 195 cm, Activity Level 1

WEIGHT LOSS PREDICTION – MEN 56 to 75 yrs

Weight Loss	Diet kcal	Present Weight (kg)							
		75	80	90	100	110	120	130	140
5 kg	1200	26	24	21	19	17	16	14	13
	1500	32	30	25	22	20	18	16	15
	1800	42	38	31	26	23	20	18	17
	2100	61	52	40	33	28	24	21	19
10 kg	1200		51	45	40	36	33	30	28
	1500		62	53	46	41	37	34	31
	1800		80	65	55	48	43	38	35
	2100		113	85	69	58	50	45	40
15 kg	1200			69	61	55	50	46	43
	1500			83	72	64	57	52	48
	1800			104	87	75	66	59	54
	2100			137	109	91	79	69	62
20 kg	1200			96	85	76	69	63	58
	1500			116	100	88	79	71	65
	1800			146	121	104	91	82	74
	2100			198	155	128	109	95	85
25 kg	1200				110	98	88	81	75
	1500				130	114	101	91	84
	1800				159	136	118	105	95
	2100				207	168	142	124	110
30 kg	1200				136	121	109	99	92
	1500				163	141	125	113	103
	1800				202	170	147	130	117
	2100				268	214	179	154	136
35 kg	1200	Values in table				146	131	119	109
	1500	are time in days				171	151	135	123
	1800	to lose weight				208	179	157	141
	2100	indicated.				266	219	187	164
40 kg	1200					173	154	140	128
	1500					204	179	160	144
	1800					251	213	186	166
	2100					327	264	224	195

Table A.35 Weight Loss Prediction: Men, 181 to 195 cm, Activity Level 2

WEIGHT LOSS PREDICTION – MEN 56 to 75 yrs

Weight Loss	Diet kcal	Present Weight (kg)							
		75	80	90	100	110	120	130	140
5 kg	1200	21	19	17	15	14	13	12	11
	1500	25	23	19	17	15	14	13	12
	1800	30	27	23	20	17	15	14	13
	2100	38	34	27	23	20	17	16	14
10 kg	1200		41	36	32	29	26	24	22
	1500		48	41	36	32	29	26	24
	1800		58	48	41	36	32	29	27
	2100		73	58	48	42	36	33	29
15 kg	1200			56	49	44	40	37	34
	1500			64	56	50	45	41	37
	1800			76	64	56	50	45	41
	2100			92	76	65	57	51	46
20 kg	1200			77	68	61	55	51	47
	1500			89	77	68	61	56	51
	1800			106	90	78	69	62	56
	2100			131	107	90	79	70	63
25 kg	1200				88	78	71	65	60
	1500				100	88	79	72	65
	1800				117	101	89	80	72
	2100				141	118	102	90	80
30 kg	1200				109	97	88	80	73
	1500				126	110	98	88	80
	1800				148	126	111	99	89
	2100				180	149	127	112	100
35 kg	1200	Values in table are time in days to lose weight indicated.				117	105	96	88
	1500					133	118	106	96
	1800					154	134	119	107
	2100					183	155	135	120
40 kg	1200					138	124	112	103
	1500					158	139	125	113
	1800					185	159	140	126
	2100					222	186	160	142

Table A.36 Weight Loss Prediction: Men, 181 to 195 cm, Activity Level 3

Appendix B Weight Loss Prediction Tables - Women

This appendix contains 24 Weight Loss Prediction Tables for Women. The
tables cover women from 18 to 75 years, with heights ranging from 150 to
180 cm, and activity levels from 0 to 4. Refer to the index in Table BB
below to find the table that's right for you.

Note, before choosing your personal Weight Loss Prediction table, you must
determine your Activity Level. (See **Table 1**. page 17)

Age	Height	Activity Levels	Table Number Page Number
18 - 35	150 to 165 cm	1 to 4	B.1 to B.4 Page 92
18 - 35	166 to 180 cm	1 to 4	B.5 to B.8 Page 96
36 - 55	150 to 165 cm	0 to 3	B.9 to B.12 Page 100
36 - 55	166 to 180 cm	0 to 3	B.13 to B.16 Page 104
56 - 75	150 to 165 cm	0 to 3	B.17 to B.20 Page 108
56 - 75	166 to 180 cm	0 to 3	B.21 to B.24 Page 112

Table BB: 24 Weight Loss Prediction Tables for Women

Once you have selected the Weight Loss Prediction table that's appropriate
for you, return to **Example 1** (page 36) for instruction on how to use the data
in the table.

WEIGHT LOSS PREDICTION – WOMEN 18 to 35 yrs

Weight Loss	Diet kcal	Present Weight (kg)							
		50	55	60	65	70	80	90	100
2	900	17	15	14	13	12	11	9	9
2	1200	25	21	19	17	15	13	11	10
2	1500	43	34	28	24	21	17	14	12
2	1800	178	82	54	41	33	24	19	15
4	900	35	31	29	26	24	21	19	17
4	1200	51	44	38	34	31	26	23	20
4	1500	92	70	58	49	43	34	29	25
4	1800		186	117	86	68	49	38	31
6	900		48	44	40	37	32	29	26
6	1200		67	59	52	47	40	35	31
6	1500		111	90	76	66	52	44	37
6	1800		330	191	136	107	75	58	48
8	900		66	60	54	50	44	39	35
8	1200		93	81	72	64	54	47	41
8	1500		157	125	104	90	71	59	51
8	1800			283	194	149	103	80	65
10	900			76	69	64	55	49	44
10	1200			104	92	82	69	59	52
10	1500			164	135	116	91	75	64
10	1800				262	197	133	102	83
15	900			120	109	100	86	76	68
15	1200			168	147	131	108	92	81
15	1500			282	226	189	145	118	100
15	1800					349	220	164	131
20	900	Values in table			154	140	119	105	93
20	1200	are time in days			211	186	151	128	112
20	1500	to lose weight			344	280	207	166	139
20	1800	indicated.					330	236	185
25	900					184	155	135	120
25	1200					251	200	167	145
25	1500						280	220	182
25	1800							322	247

Table B.1 Weight Loss Prediction: Women, 150 - 165 cm Activity Level 1

WEIGHT LOSS PREDICTION – WOMEN 18 to 35 yrs

Weight Loss	Diet kcal	Present Weight (kg)							
		50	55	60	65	70	80	90	100
2	900	15	13	12	11	10	9	8	7
2	1200	20	17	15	14	13	11	9	8
2	1500	30	25	21	18	16	13	11	10
2	1800	64	43	33	26	22	17	14	12
4	900	30	27	24	22	21	18	16	15
4	1200	41	35	31	28	25	22	19	17
4	1500	63	51	43	37	33	27	23	20
4	1800	143	93	69	55	46	35	28	24
6	900		41	37	34	32	28	25	22
6	1200		54	48	43	39	33	29	26
6	1500		80	67	57	50	41	35	30
6	1800		151	109	86	72	54	43	36
8	900		56	51	47	43	37	33	30
8	1200		75	66	59	53	45	39	34
8	1500		111	92	79	69	56	47	41
8	1800		221	155	121	99	74	59	49
10	900			65	59	55	47	42	38
10	1200			84	75	68	57	49	44
10	1500			120	102	89	71	60	51
10	1800			209	159	129	95	75	63
15	900			103	93	85	74	65	58
15	1200			136	119	107	89	77	67
15	1500			201	167	143	113	93	80
15	1800				279	218	153	120	99
20	900	Values in table			131	119	102	89	80
20	1200	are time in days			171	152	124	106	93
20	1500	to lose weight			248	208	160	131	111
20	1800	indicated.				338	224	170	138
25	900					157	133	116	103
25	1200					203	164	138	120
25	1500					289	214	172	145
25	1800						312	229	182

Table B.2 Weight Loss Prediction: Women, 150 - 165 cm Activity Level 2

WEIGHT LOSS PREDICTION – WOMEN 18 to 35 yrs

Weight Loss	Diet kcal	Present Weight (kg)							
		50	55	60	65	70	80	90	100
2	900	12	11	10	9	8	7	7	6
2	1200	15	13	12	11	10	8	7	7
2	1500	20	17	15	13	12	10	8	7
2	1800	32	25	20	17	15	12	10	9
4	900	24	22	20	18	17	15	13	12
4	1200	31	27	24	22	20	17	15	13
4	1500	42	36	31	27	24	20	17	15
4	1800	68	52	42	35	31	24	20	17
6	900		34	30	28	26	23	20	18
6	1200		42	37	33	30	26	23	20
6	1500		55	47	42	37	31	26	23
6	1800		82	66	55	47	37	31	26
8	900		46	41	38	35	30	27	24
8	1200		57	51	45	41	35	31	27
8	1500		76	65	57	51	42	35	31
8	1800		116	91	76	65	51	42	36
10	900			53	48	44	39	34	31
10	1200			65	58	53	45	39	34
10	1500			84	73	65	53	45	39
10	1800			120	98	84	65	53	45
15	900			84	76	70	60	53	47
15	1200			104	92	83	70	60	53
15	1500			138	118	104	83	70	61
15	1800			208	165	137	104	84	71
20	900	Values in table are time in days to lose weight indicated.			107	97	83	73	65
20	1200				132	118	97	83	73
20	1500				173	149	118	98	84
20	1800				253	204	149	118	99
25	900					128	108	94	84
25	1200					157	128	109	95
25	1500					203	157	128	109
25	1800					292	202	157	130

Table B.3 Weight Loss Prediction: Women, 150 - 165 cm Activity Level 3

WEIGHT LOSS PREDICTION – WOMEN 18 to 35 yrs

Weight Loss	Diet kcal	Present Weight (kg)							
		50	55	60	65	70	80	90	100
2	900	9	8	7	7	6	5	5	4
2	1200	10	9	8	8	7	6	5	5
2	1500	13	11	10	9	8	7	6	5
2	1800	16	14	12	10	9	8	6	6
4	900	18	16	15	14	13	11	10	9
4	1200	21	19	17	15	14	12	11	10
4	1500	26	23	20	18	16	14	12	10
4	1800	34	28	24	21	19	15	13	11
6	900		25	22	21	19	17	15	13
6	1200		29	26	23	21	18	16	14
6	1500		35	31	27	25	21	18	16
6	1800		44	37	32	29	23	20	17
8	900		34	31	28	26	22	20	18
8	1200		40	35	32	29	25	22	19
8	1500		48	42	37	33	28	24	21
8	1800		61	51	44	39	32	27	23
10	900			39	36	33	28	25	23
10	1200			45	41	37	32	28	25
10	1500			54	48	43	36	31	27
10	1800			66	57	50	41	34	30
15	900			62	56	51	44	39	35
15	1200			72	64	58	49	43	38
15	1500			87	76	68	56	48	42
15	1800			110	93	81	64	54	46
20	900	Values in table		79	72	61	54	48
20	1200	are time in days		91	82	69	59	52
20	1500	to lose weight		109	96	78	66	57
20	1800	indicated.		136	116	91	75	64
25	900					94	80	69	62
25	1200					109	90	77	67
25	1500					130	103	86	75
25	1800					160	121	99	83

Table B.4 Weight Loss Prediction: Women, 150 - 165 cm Activity Level 4

WEIGHT LOSS PREDICTION – WOMEN 18 to 35 yrs

Weight Loss	Diet kcal	Present Weight (kg)							
		55	60	65	70	80	90	100	110
2	900	14	13	12	11	10	9	8	7
2	1200	19	17	15	14	12	10	9	8
2	1500	28	24	21	18	15	13	11	10
2	1800	55	41	32	27	20	16	14	12
4	900	29	26	24	23	20	18	16	15
4	1200	39	34	31	28	24	21	19	17
4	1500	58	49	42	37	30	26	23	20
4	1800	120	86	67	56	42	33	28	24
6	900		40	37	34	30	27	24	22
6	1200		53	47	43	37	32	29	26
6	1500		76	65	57	47	39	34	30
6	1800		137	106	87	64	51	43	37
10	900			64	59	52	46	42	38
10	1200			82	74	63	55	49	44
10	1500			116	101	81	68	59	52
10	1800			197	157	113	89	74	63
15	900				92	80	71	64	58
15	1200				118	98	85	75	68
15	1500				163	128	106	91	80
15	1800				267	184	142	116	99
20	900					111	97	87	80
20	1200					137	118	103	92
20	1500					182	149	126	110
20	1800					270	202	163	137
25	900	Values in table				144	126	112	102
25	1200	are time in days				181	153	134	119
25	1500	to lose weight				244	196	165	143
25	1800	indicated.					273	215	179
30	900						156	139	125
30	1200						192	166	147
30	1500						249	207	178
30	1800							276	226

Table B.5 Weight Loss Prediction: Women, 166 - 180 cm Activity Level 1

WEIGHT LOSS PREDICTION – WOMEN 18 to 35 yrs

Weight Loss	Diet kcal	Present Weight (kg)							
		55	60	65	70	80	90	100	110
2	900	12	11	10	10	8	8	7	6
2	1200	16	14	13	12	10	9	8	7
2	1500	21	18	16	15	12	10	9	8
2	1800	34	27	23	19	15	13	11	9
4	900	25	23	21	20	17	15	14	13
4	1200	32	28	26	24	20	18	16	14
4	1500	44	38	33	30	25	21	18	16
4	1800	73	57	47	40	31	26	22	19
6	900		35	32	30	26	23	21	19
6	1200		44	39	36	31	27	24	22
6	1500		59	51	45	37	32	28	25
6	1800		89	73	62	48	39	33	29
10	900			55	51	45	40	36	33
10	1200			68	62	53	46	41	37
10	1500			90	80	65	55	48	42
10	1800			133	111	84	68	57	50
15	900				80	69	61	55	50
15	1200				98	82	71	63	57
15	1500				128	102	86	74	66
15	1800				183	135	107	90	77
20	900					96	84	75	68
20	1200					115	99	87	78
20	1500					144	120	103	90
20	1800					195	152	125	107
25	900	Values in table				124	109	97	88
25	1200	are time in days				151	128	112	100
25	1500	to lose weight				192	157	134	117
25	1800	indicated.				267	203	165	140
30	900						135	120	108
30	1200						161	140	124
30	1500						199	167	145
30	1800						262	209	175

Table B.6 Weight Loss Prediction: Women, 166 - 180 cm Activity Level 2

WEIGHT LOSS PREDICTION – WOMEN 18 to 35 yrs

Weight Loss	Diet kcal	Present Weight (kg)							
		55	60	65	70	80	90	100	110
2	900	10	9	9	8	7	6	6	5
2	1200	12	11	10	9	8	7	6	6
2	1500	16	14	12	11	9	8	7	6
2	1800	21	18	15	14	11	9	8	7
4	900	21	19	17	16	14	13	11	10
4	1200	25	22	20	19	16	14	13	11
4	1500	32	28	25	22	19	16	14	13
4	1800	45	37	32	28	22	19	16	14
6	900		29	26	24	21	19	17	16
6	1200		34	31	29	24	22	19	17
6	1500		43	38	34	29	25	22	19
6	1800		58	49	43	34	29	25	22
10	900			46	42	37	33	29	27
10	1200			54	49	42	37	33	30
10	1500			67	60	49	42	37	33
10	1800			88	76	60	50	43	37
15	900				66	57	50	45	41
15	1200				78	66	57	51	45
15	1500				95	78	66	57	51
15	1800				123	95	78	66	58
20	900					79	69	62	56
20	1200					91	79	70	62
20	1500					109	92	79	70
20	1800					135	109	92	80
25	900	Values in table are time in days to lose weight indicated.				102	89	80	72
25	1200					120	102	90	80
25	1500					145	120	103	90
25	1800					183	145	120	104
30	900						111	99	89
30	1200						128	112	99
30	1500						151	129	112
30	1800						185	152	129

Table B.7 Weight Loss Prediction: Women, 166 - 180 cm Activity Level 3

WEIGHT LOSS PREDICTION – WOMEN 18 to 35 yrs

Weight Loss	Diet kcal	Present Weight (kg)							
		55	60	65	70	80	90	100	110
2	900	8	7	6	6	5	5	4	4
2	1200	9	8	7	7	6	5	5	4
2	1500	10	9	8	7	6	6	5	4
2	1800	13	11	10	9	7	6	5	5
4	900	15	14	13	12	11	9	8	8
4	1200	18	16	15	13	12	10	9	8
4	1500	21	19	17	15	13	11	10	9
4	1800	26	22	20	18	15	12	11	10
6	900		21	20	18	16	14	13	12
6	1200		25	22	21	18	16	14	13
6	1500		29	26	23	20	17	15	14
6	1800		35	30	27	22	19	17	15
10	900			34	32	27	24	22	20
10	1200			39	35	30	27	24	21
10	1500			45	40	34	29	26	23
10	1800			53	47	39	33	28	25
15	900				49	43	38	34	31
15	1200				56	47	41	37	33
15	1500				64	53	46	40	36
15	1800				76	61	51	44	39
20	900					59	52	46	42
20	1200					66	57	50	45
20	1500					74	63	55	49
20	1800					86	71	61	54
25	900	Values in table are time in days to lose weight indicated.				77	67	59	54
25	1200					86	74	65	58
25	1500					98	83	71	63
25	1800					114	93	79	69
30	900						83	74	66
30	1200						92	81	72
30	1500						104	89	78
30	1800						118	100	86

Table B.8 Weight Loss Prediction: Women, 166 - 180 cm Activity Level 4

WEIGHT LOSS PREDICTION – WOMEN 36 to 55 yrs

Weight Loss	Diet kcal	Present Weight (kg)							
		50	55	60	65	70	80	90	100
2	900	20	18	16	15	14	12	11	10
2	1200	30	25	22	20	18	15	13	12
2	1500	63	46	36	30	26	20	17	14
2	1800		238	100	64	47	32	24	19
4	900	40	36	33	30	28	24	21	19
4	1200	62	52	46	40	36	30	26	23
4	1500	137	97	76	62	53	42	34	29
4	1800			229	139	100	65	49	39
6	900		55	50	45	42	37	32	29
6	1200		81	70	62	56	46	40	35
6	1500		156	119	97	83	64	52	45
6	1800				228	160	102	75	60
8	900		75	68	62	57	49	44	39
8	1200		112	96	85	76	63	54	48
8	1500		224	168	135	114	87	71	60
8	1800				341	229	141	103	82
10	900			86	79	72	63	55	50
10	1200			124	109	97	80	69	60
10	1500			222	177	147	112	91	77
10	1800					311	184	133	105
15	900			137	124	113	97	86	77
15	1200			204	175	155	126	107	94
15	1500				302	244	179	143	120
15	1800						313	216	167
20	900	Values in table			175	159	135	118	105
20	1200	are time in days			255	221	177	149	129
20	1500	to lose weight					259	202	167
20	1800	indicated.						317	238
25	900					210	176	153	135
25	1200					301	235	195	167
25	1500							270	220
25	1800								321

Table B.9 Weight Loss Prediction: Women, 150 - 165 cm Activity Level 0

WEIGHT LOSS PREDICTION – WOMEN 36 to 55 yrs

Weight Loss	Diet kcal	Present Weight (kg)							
		50	55	60	65	70	80	90	100
2	900	18	16	15	13	12	11	10	9
2	1200	26	23	20	18	16	14	12	10
2	1500	49	37	30	26	22	18	15	13
2	1800		109	65	47	37	26	20	16
4	900	37	33	30	27	25	22	20	18
4	1200	55	47	41	36	33	27	24	21
4	1500	105	79	63	53	46	36	30	26
4	1800		259	142	99	76	53	41	33
6	900		51	46	42	39	34	30	27
6	1200		72	63	55	50	42	36	32
6	1500		125	99	82	71	55	46	39
6	1800			238	159	121	82	63	51
8	900		69	62	57	52	45	40	36
8	1200		99	86	76	68	57	49	43
8	1500		177	138	114	97	76	62	53
8	1800			230	170	113	86	70	
10	900			80	72	67	58	51	46
10	1200			110	97	87	72	62	55
10	1500			182	148	125	97	79	68
10	1800			315	226	147	110	89	
15	900			126	114	104	90	79	71
15	1200			180	156	138	113	97	85
15	1500			318	249	206	155	125	106
15	1800					245	177	140	
20	900	Values in table			161	146	124	109	97
20	1200	are time in days			226	197	159	134	117
20	1500	to lose weight				307	222	176	147
20	1800	indicated.						257	199
25	900					193	162	141	125
25	1200					267	211	175	151
25	1500						303	234	193
25	1800								266

Table B.10 Weight Loss Prediction: Women, 150 - 165 cm Activity Level 1

WEIGHT LOSS PREDICTION – WOMEN 36 to 55 yrs

Weight Loss	Diet kcal	Present Weight (kg)							
		50	55	60	65	70	80	90	100
2	900	15	14	12	11	11	9	8	7
2	1200	21	18	16	14	13	11	10	9
2	1500	33	26	22	19	17	14	12	10
2	1800	78	49	36	29	24	18	15	12
4	900	31	28	25	23	22	19	17	15
4	1200	43	37	33	29	27	23	20	17
4	1500	69	55	46	39	35	28	24	21
4	1800	180	107	77	60	50	37	30	25
6	900		43	39	36	33	29	25	23
6	1200		57	50	45	41	34	30	26
6	1500		87	71	61	53	43	36	31
6	1800		177	123	95	78	57	46	38
8	900		59	53	48	45	39	34	31
8	1200		79	69	61	55	47	40	36
8	1500		121	99	84	73	58	49	42
8	1800		265	176	133	108	79	62	52
10	900			68	62	57	49	43	39
10	1200			89	78	71	59	51	45
10	1500			129	109	94	75	62	54
10	1800			240	177	141	101	80	66
15	900			107	97	89	76	67	60
15	1200			143	126	112	93	79	70
15	1500			218	179	152	119	98	83
15	1800				317	240	165	127	104
20	900	Values in table			137	124	106	92	82
20	1200	are time in days			180	159	130	110	96
20	1500	to lose weight			268	223	169	137	116
20	1800	indicated.					242	181	146
25	900					164	138	119	106
25	1200					214	171	144	125
25	1500					312	227	181	151
25	1800						342	245	193

Table B.11 Weight Loss Prediction: Women, 150 - 165 cm Activity Level 2

WEIGHT LOSS PREDICTION – WOMEN 36 to 55 yrs

Weight Loss	Diet kcal	Present Weight (kg)							
		50	55	60	65	70	80	90	100
2	900	12	11	10	9	9	8	7	6
2	1200	16	14	12	11	10	9	8	7
2	1500	22	18	16	14	12	10	9	8
2	1800	35	27	22	18	16	12	10	9
4	900	25	23	21	19	17	15	14	12
4	1200	32	28	25	23	21	18	15	14
4	1500	45	38	32	28	25	21	18	16
4	1800	75	56	45	37	32	25	21	18
6	900		35	31	29	27	23	21	18
6	1200		43	39	35	31	27	23	21
6	1500		58	50	43	39	32	27	24
6	1800		89	70	58	50	39	32	27
8	900		47	43	39	36	31	28	25
8	1200		60	53	47	43	36	32	28
8	1500		81	68	59	53	43	37	32
8	1800		126	98	81	69	53	44	37
10	900			55	50	46	40	35	31
10	1200			67	60	55	46	40	35
10	1500			89	77	68	55	46	40
10	1800			129	105	89	68	56	47
15	900			86	78	72	62	54	48
15	1200			109	96	86	72	62	55
15	1500			146	124	108	87	73	63
15	1800			227	177	146	109	88	74
20	900	Values in table		110	100	85	75	66
20	1200	are time in days		137	122	101	86	75
20	1500	to lose weight		182	156	122	101	87
20	1800	indicated.		274	218	157	124	103
25	900					132	111	97	86
25	1200					163	132	112	97
25	1500					214	163	133	113
25	1800					315	214	165	135

Table B.12 Weight Loss Prediction: Women, 150 - 165 cm Activity Level 3

WEIGHT LOSS PREDICTION – WOMEN 36 to 55 yrs

Weight Loss	Diet kcal	Present Weight (kg)							
		55	60	65	70	80	90	100	110
2	900	16	15	14	13	11	10	9	8
2	1200	23	20	18	17	14	12	11	10
2	1500	39	32	27	23	19	16	13	12
2	1800	126	72	51	40	28	22	18	15
4	900	34	31	28	26	23	20	18	17
4	1200	48	42	37	34	29	25	22	20
4	1500	82	66	56	48	38	32	27	24
4	1800	306	159	109	83	57	44	36	31
6	900		47	43	40	35	31	28	26
6	1200		64	57	52	44	38	33	30
6	1500		104	86	74	58	48	42	37
6	1800		268	175	131	89	68	55	47
10	900			74	68	59	53	48	43
10	1200			100	90	75	65	57	51
10	1500			155	132	102	84	71	63
10	1800				247	159	119	95	80
15	900				107	92	81	73	67
15	1200				143	118	101	88	79
15	1500				216	163	132	111	97
15	1800					266	191	151	126
20	900					128	112	100	91
20	1200					165	140	122	108
20	1500					233	186	155	134
20	1800						278	214	176
25	900	Values in table				166	145	129	117
25	1200	are time in days				218	182	158	140
25	1500	to lose weight				318	247	203	174
25	1800	indicated.						287	231
30	900							180	160	144
30	1200						230	197	173
30	1500						317	257	218
30	1800								294

Table B.13 Weight Loss Prediction: Women, 166 - 180 cm Activity Level 0

WEIGHT LOSS PREDICTION – WOMEN 36 to 55 yrs

Weight Loss	Diet kcal	Present Weight (kg)							
		55	60	65	70	80	90	100	110
2	900	15	14	13	12	10	9	8	8
2	1200	21	18	17	15	13	11	10	9
2	1500	33	27	23	20	16	14	12	11
2	1800	77	52	39	32	23	18	15	13
4	900	31	28	26	24	21	19	17	16
4	1200	43	38	34	31	26	23	20	18
4	1500	69	56	48	42	34	28	24	22
4	1800	174	112	83	66	48	37	31	27
6	900		43	40	37	32	29	26	24
6	1200		58	52	47	39	34	30	27
6	1500		88	74	64	51	43	37	33
6	1800		182	131	104	73	57	47	40
10	900			69	63	55	49	44	40
10	1200			90	81	68	59	52	47
10	1500			133	114	89	74	64	56
10	1800			252	191	131	100	82	69
15	900				99	85	75	68	62
15	1200				129	107	91	80	72
15	1500				186	142	116	99	87
15	1800				336	215	160	129	109
20	900					118	104	93	84
20	1200					149	127	111	99
20	1500					203	163	138	119
20	1800					321	231	182	151
25	900	Values in table				154	134	119	108
25	1200	are time in days				197	165	143	127
25	1500	to lose weight				275	216	180	155
25	1800	indicated.					315	242	199
30	900						167	148	133
30	1200						208	179	157
30	1500						277	227	193
30	1800							313	251

Table B.14 Weight Loss Prediction: Women, 166 - 180 cm Activity Level 1

WEIGHT LOSS PREDICTION – WOMEN 36 to 55 yrs

Weight Loss	Diet kcal	Present Weight (kg)							
		55	60	65	70	80	90	100	110
2	900	13	12	11	10	9	8	7	7
2	1200	17	15	14	12	11	9	8	7
2	1500	24	20	18	16	13	11	10	9
2	1800	42	32	26	22	17	14	12	10
4	900	27	24	22	21	18	16	15	13
4	1200	35	31	28	25	21	19	17	15
4	1500	50	42	37	32	26	22	20	17
4	1800	89	67	54	45	34	28	24	21
6	900		37	34	31	27	24	22	20
6	1200		47	42	39	33	29	25	23
6	1500		65	56	50	40	34	30	26
6	1800		106	84	70	53	43	36	31
10	900			59	54	47	42	38	34
10	1200			74	67	56	49	43	39
10	1500			100	87	70	59	51	45
10	1800			155	126	93	74	62	54
15	900				85	73	64	58	53
15	1200				106	88	76	67	60
15	1500				141	111	92	79	70
15	1800				213	151	118	97	83
20	900					101	89	79	72
20	1200					123	105	92	82
20	1500					158	129	110	96
20	1800					220	168	136	116
25	900	Values in table				132	115	102	92
25	1200	are time in days				162	137	119	106
25	1500	to lose weight				211	170	143	124
25	1800	indicated.				306	225	180	151
30	900						143	126	113
30	1200						172	148	131
30	1500						217	180	155
30	1800						294	230	190

Table B.15 Weight Loss Prediction: Women, 166 - 180 cm Activity Level 2

WEIGHT LOSS PREDICTION – WOMEN 36 to 55 yrs

Weight Loss	Diet kcal	Present Weight (kg)							
		55	60	65	70	80	90	100	110
2	900	11	10	9	8	7	6	6	5
2	1200	13	12	11	10	8	7	7	6
2	1500	17	15	13	12	10	8	7	7
2	1800	24	20	17	15	12	10	8	7
4	900	22	20	18	17	15	13	12	11
4	1200	27	24	22	20	17	15	13	12
4	1500	35	30	27	24	20	17	15	13
4	1800	51	41	35	30	24	20	17	15
6	900		30	28	26	22	20	18	16
6	1200		37	33	30	26	23	20	18
6	1500		47	41	37	30	26	23	20
6	1800		64	54	47	37	31	26	23
10	900			48	44	38	34	31	28
10	1200			58	52	44	39	34	31
10	1500			72	64	52	45	39	35
10	1800			97	83	64	53	45	39
15	900				69	60	52	47	43
15	1200				83	69	60	53	47
15	1500				102	83	70	60	53
15	1800				135	103	83	70	61
20	900					82	72	65	58
20	1200					97	83	73	65
20	1500					117	97	83	73
20	1800					147	117	98	84
25	900	Values in table are time in days to lose weight indicated.				107	94	83	75
25	1200					127	108	94	84
25	1500					155	127	109	95
25	1800					200	156	128	110
30	900						116	103	92
30	1200						135	117	104
30	1500						161	136	118
30	1800						200	162	137

Table B.16 Weight Loss Prediction: Women, 166 - 180 cm Activity Level 3

WEIGHT LOSS PREDICTION – WOMEN 56 to 75 yrs

Weight Loss	Diet kcal	Present Weight (kg)							
		50	55	60	65	70	80	90	100
2	900	22	19	17	16	15	13	11	10
2	1200	35	29	25	22	20	16	14	12
2	1500	88	58	44	36	30	23	19	16
2	1800			196	95	63	38	28	22
4	900	44	39	35	32	30	26	23	21
4	1200	72	60	51	45	40	33	29	25
4	1500	199	126	93	74	62	47	38	32
4	1800				214	136	80	57	45
6	900		60	54	49	45	39	35	31
6	1200		93	79	69	62	51	43	38
6	1500		205	148	116	96	72	58	49
6	1800					222	125	88	69
8	900		82	74	67	61	53	47	42
8	1200		129	109	95	84	69	59	51
8	1500		303	210	162	133	99	79	66
8	1800					327	175	121	94
10	900			94	85	78	67	59	53
10	1200			141	122	108	88	75	65
10	1500			283	214	173	127	101	84
10	1800						231	157	120
15	900			150	135	123	104	91	82
15	1200			233	198	172	138	116	101
15	1500					293	206	160	132
15	1800							259	192
20	900	Values in table			191	172	145	126	112
20	1200	are time in days			290	248	195	162	140
20	1500	to lose weight					300	228	185
20	1800	indicated.							277
25	900					228	190	164	144
25	1200					341	260	213	181
25	1500							307	245
25	1800								

Table B.17 Weight Loss Prediction: Women, 150 - 165 cm Activity Level 0

WEIGHT LOSS PREDICTION – WOMEN 56 to 75 yrs

Weight Loss	Diet kcal	Present Weight (kg)							
		50	55	60	65	70	80	90	100
2	900	20	18	16	14	13	12	10	9
2	1200	30	25	22	19	17	15	13	11
2	1500	63	45	36	29	25	20	16	14
2	1800		225	95	61	45	30	23	18
4	900	40	36	32	29	27	24	21	19
4	1200	62	52	45	40	36	30	26	23
4	1500	138	96	75	61	52	40	33	28
4	1800			218	132	95	62	46	37
6	900		55	49	45	41	36	32	29
6	1200		81	70	61	55	45	39	34
6	1500		155	117	95	80	62	50	43
6	1800				217	152	97	71	57
8	900		75	67	61	56	48	43	38
8	1200		112	96	84	75	62	53	46
8	1500		223	165	132	111	84	68	58
8	1800				325	218	134	98	78
10	900			86	78	71	61	54	49
10	1200			123	107	95	78	67	58
10	1500			220	173	144	108	87	74
10	1800					295	175	126	99
15	900			137	123	112	96	84	75
15	1200			203	174	152	123	104	91
15	1500				298	239	174	138	115
15	1800						298	205	158
20	900	Values in table		174	157	133	116	103	
20	1200	are time in days		253	219	174	145	125	
20	1500	to lose weight				252	195	161	
20	1800	indicated.					301	225	
25	900					208	174	150	132
25	1200					298	231	190	163
25	1500						347	261	212
25	1800							304	

Table B.18 Weight Loss Prediction: Women, 150 - 165 cm Activity Level 1

WEIGHT LOSS PREDICTION – WOMEN 56 to 75 yrs

Weight Loss	Diet kcal	Present Weight (kg)							
		50	55	60	65	70	80	90	100
2	900	16	15	13	12	11	10	9	8
2	1200	23	20	17	15	14	12	10	9
2	1500	39	30	25	21	19	15	13	11
2	1800	121	64	44	34	28	20	16	13
4	900	34	30	27	25	23	20	18	16
4	1200	48	41	36	32	29	24	21	18
4	1500	82	63	52	44	38	30	25	22
4	1800	309	143	95	71	57	42	33	27
6	900		46	41	38	35	30	27	24
6	1200		63	55	49	44	37	32	28
6	1500		100	81	68	59	47	39	33
6	1800		246	154	113	90	64	50	41
8	900		63	56	51	47	41	36	32
8	1200		87	75	66	60	50	43	38
8	1500		141	112	94	81	64	53	45
8	1800			225	160	125	88	68	56
10	900			72	65	60	52	46	41
10	1200			97	85	76	63	54	48
10	1500			147	122	104	81	67	57
10	1800			314	215	165	114	88	72
15	900			115	103	94	80	71	63
15	1200			157	137	121	99	85	74
15	1500			253	203	170	130	105	89
15	1800					288	187	140	113
20	900	Values in table			146	132	112	97	86
20	1200	are time in days			197	173	139	117	102
20	1500	to lose weight			309	251	185	148	124
20	1800	indicated.					279	201	159
25	900					175	146	126	111
25	1200					234	184	153	132
25	1500						251	197	163
25	1800							275	212

Table B.19 Weight Loss Prediction: Women, 150 - 165 cm Activity Level 2

WEIGHT LOSS PREDICTION – WOMEN 56 to 75 yrs

Weight Loss	Diet kcal	Present Weight (kg)							
		50	55	60	65	70	80	90	100
2	900	13	12	11	10	9	8	7	6
2	1200	17	15	13	12	11	9	8	7
2	1500	24	20	17	15	13	11	9	8
2	1800	42	30	24	20	17	13	11	9
4	900	27	24	22	20	18	16	14	13
4	1200	35	30	27	24	22	18	16	14
4	1500	50	41	35	30	27	22	19	16
4	1800	90	64	50	41	35	27	22	19
6	900		37	33	30	28	24	21	19
6	1200		47	41	37	33	28	24	22
6	1500		64	54	47	41	34	28	25
6	1800		103	79	65	55	42	34	29
8	900		50	45	41	38	33	29	26
8	1200		64	56	50	45	38	33	29
8	1500		89	75	64	57	46	39	33
8	1800		148	111	90	75	57	46	39
10	900			57	52	48	41	36	33
10	1200			72	64	58	48	42	37
10	1500			97	83	73	58	49	42
10	1800			147	117	97	73	59	50
15	900			91	82	75	64	56	50
15	1200			116	102	92	76	65	57
15	1500			161	135	117	92	77	66
15	1800			266	200	162	118	94	78
20	900	Values in table		116	106	89	78	69
20	1200	are time in days		147	130	106	90	79
20	1500	to lose weight		200	169	131	107	91
20	1800	indicated.		318	245	171	133	109
25	900					139	117	101	89
25	1200					174	140	118	102
25	1500					234	175	141	119
25	1800						235	178	144

Table B.20 Weight Loss Prediction: Women, 150 - 165 cm Activity Level 3

WEIGHT LOSS PREDICTION – WOMEN 56 to 75 yrs

Weight Loss	Diet kcal	Present Weight (kg)							
		55	60	65	70	80	90	100	110
2	900	18	16	15	14	12	11	10	9
2	1200	26	23	20	18	15	13	12	11
2	1500	48	38	31	27	21	17	15	13
2	1800	314	111	69	50	33	25	20	17
4	900	37	33	30	28	24	22	20	18
4	1200	54	47	41	37	31	27	24	21
4	1500	102	79	65	55	43	35	30	26
4	1800		261	150	106	68	50	40	34
6	900		51	46	43	37	33	30	27
6	1200		72	63	57	47	41	36	32
6	1500		124	101	85	65	53	45	40
6	1800			249	170	106	78	62	52
10	900			80	73	63	56	50	46
10	1200			111	99	82	70	61	55
10	1500			183	152	114	93	78	68
10	1800				333	192	137	108	89
15	900				115	99	87	78	71
15	1200				158	128	109	95	85
15	1500				253	184	146	122	105
15	1800					329	224	172	140
20	900					137	120	107	96
20	1200					181	151	131	116
20	1500					267	207	171	146
20	1800						330	245	197
25	900	Values in table				179	155	137	124
25	1200	are time in days				240	198	170	150
25	1500	to lose weight					277	224	190
25	1800	indicated.						332	261
30	900						193	170	152
30	1200						250	213	186
30	1500							285	238
30	1800								334

Table B.21 Weight Loss Prediction: Women, 166 - 180 cm Activity Level 0

WEIGHT LOSS PREDICTION – WOMEN 56 to 75 yrs

Weight Loss	Diet kcal	Present Weight (kg)							
		55	60	65	70	80	90	100	110
2	900	16	15	14	13	11	10	9	8
2	1200	23	20	18	16	14	12	11	10
2	1500	39	31	26	23	18	15	13	11
2	1800	122	70	49	38	26	20	17	14
4	900	34	30	28	26	22	20	18	16
4	1200	48	41	37	33	28	24	21	19
4	1500	82	65	54	47	37	31	26	23
4	1800	299	153	105	80	55	42	34	29
6	900		47	43	39	34	30	27	25
6	1200		64	57	51	43	37	32	29
6	1500		102	85	72	57	47	40	35
6	1800		259	169	126	85	64	52	44
10	900			74	68	58	52	46	42
10	1200			99	89	73	63	55	50
10	1500			153	129	99	81	69	60
10	1800			338	238	152	113	91	76
15	900				106	91	80	71	65
15	1200				141	115	98	86	76
15	1500				212	158	128	107	93
15	1800					254	183	144	119
20	900					126	110	98	89
20	1200					162	136	118	105
20	1500					228	180	150	129
20	1800						265	204	167
25	900	Values in table				164	142	126	114
25	1200	are time in days				215	178	154	135
25	1500	to lose weight				311	239	196	167
25	1800	indicated.						273	220
30	900						177	156	140
30	1200						225	192	168
30	1500						309	249	210
30	1800								280

Table B.22 Weight Loss Prediction: Women, 166 - 180 cm Activity Level 1

WEIGHT LOSS PREDICTION – WOMEN 56 to 75 yrs

Weight Loss	Diet kcal	Present Weight (kg)							
		55	60	65	70	80	90	100	110
2	900	14	13	12	11	9	8	8	7
2	1200	18	16	15	13	11	10	9	8
2	1500	27	23	20	17	14	12	10	9
2	1800	52	38	30	25	19	15	13	11
4	900	28	26	24	22	19	17	15	14
4	1200	38	33	30	27	23	20	18	16
4	1500	57	47	40	35	29	24	21	18
4	1800	113	80	62	51	38	30	25	22
6	900		39	36	33	29	26	23	21
6	1200		51	46	41	35	30	27	24
6	1500		73	62	54	44	37	32	28
6	1800		129	98	80	59	47	39	33
10	900			62	57	50	44	39	36
10	1200			80	72	60	52	46	41
10	1500			111	96	76	63	54	48
10	1800			183	145	104	81	67	57
15	900				90	77	68	61	55
15	1200				114	94	80	71	63
15	1500				156	121	99	85	74
15	1800				249	169	129	106	89
20	900					107	93	83	75
20	1200					132	112	97	86
20	1500					172	139	117	102
20	1800					249	185	148	124
25	900	Values in table				139	121	107	96
25	1200	are time in days				174	146	126	111
25	1500	to lose weight				232	184	154	132
25	1800	indicated.					250	197	163
30	900						151	133	119
30	1200						183	157	138
30	1500						235	193	165
30	1800						330	252	206

Table B.23 Weight Loss Prediction: Women, 166 - 180 cm Activity Level 2

WEIGHT LOSS PREDICTION – WOMEN 56 to 75 yrs

Weight Loss	Diet kcal	Present Weight (kg)							
		55	60	65	70	80	90	100	110
2	900	11	10	9	9	8	7	6	6
2	1200	14	12	11	10	9	8	7	6
2	1500	18	16	14	12	10	9	8	7
2	1800	27	22	18	16	13	10	9	8
4	900	23	21	19	18	15	14	12	11
4	1200	29	25	23	21	18	16	14	12
4	1500	38	33	29	26	21	18	16	14
4	1800	58	46	38	33	26	21	18	16
6	900		32	29	27	23	21	19	17
6	1200		39	35	32	27	24	21	19
6	1500		51	44	39	32	27	24	21
6	1800		72	59	51	40	33	28	24
10	900			50	46	40	35	32	29
10	1200			61	55	47	40	36	32
10	1500			78	69	56	47	41	36
10	1800			107	90	69	56	48	41
15	900				72	62	55	49	44
15	1200				87	73	63	55	49
15	1500				110	88	73	63	56
15	1800				149	111	89	74	64
20	900					86	75	67	61
20	1200					102	87	76	68
20	1500					124	103	88	77
20	1800					160	125	104	89
25	900	Values in table				112	98	86	78
25	1200	are time in days				134	113	98	87
25	1500	to lose weight				166	135	114	99
25	1800	indicated.				218	167	136	116
30	900						122	107	96
30	1200						142	123	108
30	1500						171	143	124
30	1800						216	173	145

Table B.24 Weight Loss Prediction: Women, 166 - 180 cm Activity Level 3

Appendix C Weight Maintenance Tables - Men

This appendix contains nine Weight Maintenance Tables for Men. The tables cover men from 18 to 75 years, with heights ranging from 150 to 195 cm, and activity levels from 0 to 4. Refer to the index shown in Table CC below to find the table that's right for you. Before choosing your personal Weight Maintenance table, determine your Activity Level (**Table 1** page 18).

Age	Height	Activity Levels	Table Number Page Number
18 - 35	150 to 165 cm	1 to 4	C.1 page 117
18 - 35	166 to 180 cm	1 to 4	C.2 page 118
18 - 35	181 to 195 cm	1 to 4	C.3 page 119
36 - 55	150 to 165 cm	0 to 3	C.4 page 120
36 - 55	166 to 180 cm	0 to 3	C.5 page 121
36 - 55	181 to 195 cm	0 to 3	C.6 page 122
56 - 75	150 to 165 cm	0 to 3	C.7 page 123
56 - 75	166 to 180 cm	0 to 3	C.8 page 124
56 - 75	181 to 195 cm	0 to 3	C.9 page 125

Table CC: 9 Weight Maintenance Tables for Men

Once you have selected the Weight Maintenance table that's appropriate for you, return to **Example 2** (page 44) for instruction on how to use the data in the table.

WEIGHT MAINTENANCE – MEN

Age: 18 to 35 yrs **Height: 150 to 165 cm**

Weight (kg)	ACTIVITY				
	Level 0	Level 1	Level 2	Level 3	Level 4
46	1865	1937	2096	2346	2825
48	1910	1984	2150	2412	2911
50	1954	2031	2204	2476	2997
52	1997	2077	2257	2540	3082
54	2039	2123	2310	2604	3166
56	2081	2168	2362	2667	3250
58	2123	2213	2414	2729	3333
60	2164	2257	2465	2791	3416
62	2205	2301	2515	2853	3498
64	2245	2344	2566	2914	3580
66	2285	2387	2616	2975	3662
68	2324	2430	2665	3035	3743
70	2364	2472	2714	3095	3824
75	2460	2576	2836	3244	4024
80	2554	2678	2955	3391	4223
85	2647	2779	3073	3535	4420
90	2738	2877	3189	3679	4615
95	2827	2975	3303	3821	4809
100	2916	3070	3417	3961	5002
105	3003	3165	3529	4100	5193
110	3088	3259	3639	4238	5383
115	3173	3351	3749	4375	5572

Values in table are kcal per day.

Table C.1 Maintenance: Men 18 - 35, 150 to 165 cm

WEIGHT MAINTENANCE – MEN

Age: 18 to 35 yrs   **Height: 166 to 180 cm**

Weight (kg)	ACTIVITY				
	Level 0	Level 1	Level 2	Level 3	Level 4
56	2192	2279	2473	2778	3360
58	2235	2325	2526	2842	3445
60	2278	2371	2579	2905	3530
62	2320	2416	2631	2969	3614
64	2362	2461	2683	3031	3697
66	2404	2506	2734	3094	3780
68	2445	2550	2785	3156	3863
70	2485	2594	2836	3217	3945
72	2525	2637	2886	3278	4027
74	2565	2680	2936	3339	4109
76	2605	2723	2986	3399	4190
78	2644	2765	3035	3460	4271
80	2683	2807	3084	3519	4352
85	2779	2911	3205	3668	4552
90	2873	3013	3324	3814	4751
95	2966	3113	3442	3959	4948
100	3057	3212	3558	4103	5143
105	3147	3310	3673	4245	5337
110	3236	3406	3787	4386	5530
115	3323	3501	3899	4526	5722
120	3410	3596	4011	4664	5913
125	3495	3689	4121	4802	6103

Values in table are kcal per day.

Table C.2 Maintenance: Men 18 - 35, 166 to 180 cm

WEIGHT MAINTENANCE – MEN

Age: 18 to 35 yrs   **Height: 181 to 195 cm**

Weight (kg)	ACTIVITY				
	Level 0	Level 1	Level 2	Level 3	Level 4
66	2504	2606	2835	3194	3881
68	2546	2652	2887	3257	3965
70	2588	2697	2939	3320	4048
72	2630	2741	2990	3382	4132
74	2671	2785	3041	3444	4214
76	2711	2829	3092	3506	4297
78	2752	2873	3143	3567	4379
80	2792	2916	3193	3628	4461
82	2832	2959	3242	3689	4542
84	2871	3001	3292	3749	4623
86	2910	3043	3341	3809	4704
88	2949	3085	3390	3869	4785
90	2988	3127	3439	3929	4865
95	3083	3230	3559	4076	5065
100	3177	3332	3678	4222	5263
105	3269	3432	3795	4367	5460
110	3360	3531	3912	4510	5655
115	3450	3629	4026	4653	5849
120	3539	3725	4140	4794	6042
125	3627	3821	4253	4934	6235
130	3714	3915	4365	5073	6426
135	3800	4009	4476	5211	6616

Values in table are kcal per day.

Table C.3 Maintenance: Men 18 - 35, 181 to 195 cm

WEIGHT MAINTENANCE – MEN
Age: 36 to 55 yrs   Height: 150 to 165 cm

Weight (kg)	ACTIVITY			
	Level 0	Level 1	Level 2	Level 3
46	1785	1856	2015	2266
48	1828	1902	2068	2330
50	1870	1948	2121	2393
52	1912	1992	2172	2455
54	1953	2037	2224	2518
56	1994	2081	2274	2579
58	2034	2124	2325	2640
60	2074	2167	2375	2701
62	2113	2209	2424	2762
64	2152	2251	2473	2821
66	2191	2293	2522	2881
68	2229	2335	2570	2940
70	2267	2376	2618	2999
75	2361	2477	2736	3145
80	2452	2576	2853	3289
85	2542	2674	2968	3431
90	2631	2770	3081	3572
95	2718	2865	3194	3711
100	2803	2958	3304	3849
105	2888	3051	3414	3986
110	2972	3142	3523	4122
115	3054	3232	3630	4256

Values in table are kcal per day.

Table C.4 Maintenance: Men 36 - 55, 150 to 165 cm

WEIGHT MAINTENANCE – MEN
Age: 36 to 55 yrs   Height: 166 to 180 cm

Weight (kg)	ACTIVITY			
	Level 0	Level 1	Level 2	Level 3
56	2060	2147	2341	2646
58	2101	2191	2392	2708
60	2142	2235	2443	2770
62	2183	2279	2493	2831
64	2223	2322	2543	2892
66	2262	2364	2593	2952
68	2301	2407	2642	3012
70	2340	2449	2691	3072
72	2379	2490	2739	3131
74	2417	2531	2788	3190
76	2455	2572	2835	3249
78	2492	2613	2883	3308
80	2530	2653	2930	3366
85	2621	2753	3047	3510
90	2712	2851	3163	3653
95	2801	2948	3277	3794
100	2888	3043	3389	3934
105	2975	3137	3501	4072
110	3060	3230	3611	4210
115	3144	3322	3720	4346
120	3227	3413	3829	4482
125	3310	3503	3936	4617

Values in table are kcal per day.

Table C.5 Maintenance: Men 36 - 55, 166 to 180 cm

WEIGHT MAINTENANCE – MEN

Age: 36 to 55 yrs **Height: 181 to 195 cm**

Weight (kg)	ACTIVITY			
	Level 0	Level 1	Level 2	Level 3
66	2404	2506	2734	3094
68	2445	2550	2785	3156
70	2485	2594	2836	3217
72	2525	2637	2886	3278
74	2565	2680	2936	3339
76	2605	2723	2986	3399
78	2644	2765	3035	3460
80	2683	2807	3084	3519
82	2722	2849	3132	3579
84	2760	2890	3181	3638
86	2798	2931	3229	3697
88	2836	2972	3277	3756
90	2873	3013	3324	3814
95	2966	3113	3442	3959
100	3057	3212	3558	4103
105	3147	3310	3673	4245
110	3236	3406	3787	4386
115	3323	3501	3899	4526
120	3410	3596	4011	4664
125	3495	3689	4121	4802
130	3580	3781	4231	4939
135	3664	3873	4340	5075

Values in table are kcal per day.

Table C.6 Maintenance: Men 36 - 55, 181 to 195 cm

WEIGHT MAINTENANCE – MEN

Age: 56 to 75 yrs **Height: 150 to 165 cm**

Weight (kg)	ACTIVITY			
	Level 0	Level 1	Level 2	Level 3
46	1693	1765	1924	2174
48	1735	1809	1975	2236
50	1775	1853	2026	2298
52	1815	1896	2076	2359
54	1855	1939	2126	2420
56	1894	1981	2175	2480
58	1933	2023	2224	2539
60	1971	2064	2272	2599
62	2009	2105	2320	2658
64	2047	2146	2368	2716
66	2084	2186	2415	2774
68	2121	2226	2462	2832
70	2158	2266	2508	2890
75	2248	2364	2624	3032
80	2336	2460	2737	3173
85	2423	2555	2849	3312
90	2509	2648	2960	3450
95	2593	2740	3069	3586
100	2676	2831	3177	3722
105	2758	2921	3284	3856
110	2839	3009	3390	3989
115	2919	3097	3495	4121

Values in table are kcal per day.

Table C.7 Maintenance: Men 56 - 75, 150 to 165 cm

123

WEIGHT MAINTENANCE – MEN

Age: 56 to 75 yrs   **Height: 166 to 180 cm**

Weight (kg)	ACTIVITY			
	Level 0	Level 1	Level 2	Level 3
56	1958	2045	2239	2544
58	1998	2088	2288	2604
60	2037	2130	2338	2664
62	2076	2172	2387	2724
64	2115	2214	2435	2784
66	2153	2255	2483	2843
68	2190	2296	2531	2901
70	2228	2336	2579	2960
72	2265	2377	2626	3018
74	2302	2417	2673	3076
76	2338	2456	2719	3133
78	2375	2496	2765	3190
80	2411	2535	2811	3247
85	2500	2631	2925	3388
90	2587	2726	3038	3528
95	2673	2820	3149	3666
100	2758	2913	3259	3803
105	2841	3004	3367	3939
110	2924	3094	3475	4074
115	3006	3184	3582	4208
120	3086	3272	3687	4341
125	3166	3360	3792	4473

Values in table are kcal per day.

Table C.8 Maintenance: Men 56 - 75, 166 to 180 cm

WEIGHT MAINTENANCE – MEN

Age: 56 to 75 yrs   **Height: 181 to 195 cm**

Weight (kg)	ACTIVITY			
	Level 0	Level 1	Level 2	Level 3
66	2285	2387	2616	2975
68	2324	2430	2665	3035
70	2364	2472	2714	3095
72	2402	2514	2763	3155
74	2441	2555	2812	3214
76	2479	2597	2860	3273
78	2517	2638	2907	3332
80	2554	2678	2955	3391
82	2592	2719	3002	3449
84	2628	2759	3049	3507
86	2665	2798	3096	3564
88	2702	2838	3142	3622
90	2738	2877	3189	3679
95	2827	2975	3303	3821
100	2916	3070	3417	3961
105	3003	3165	3529	4100
110	3088	3259	3639	4238
115	3173	3351	3749	4375
120	3257	3443	3858	4511
125	3340	3533	3966	4646
130	3422	3623	4073	4781
135	3503	3712	4179	4914

Values in table are kcal per day.

Table C.9 Maintenance: Men 56 - 75 yrs, 181 to 195 cm

Appendix D Weight Maintenance Tables - Women

This appendix contains six Weight Maintenance Tables for Women. The tables cover women from 18 to 75 years, with heights ranging from 150 to 180 cm, and activity levels from 0 to 4. Refer to the index shown in Table DD below to find the table that's right for you.

Before choosing your personal Weight Maintenance table, you must determine your Activity Level. (See **Table 1**. page 18)

Age	Height	Activity Levels	Table Number Page number
18 - 35	150 to 165 cm	1 to 4	D.1 page 127
18 - 35	166 to 180 cm	1 to 4	D.2 page 128
36 - 55	150 to 165 cm	0 to 3	D.3 page 129
36 - 55	166 to 180 cm	0 to 3	D.4 page 130
56 - 75	150 to 165 cm	0 to 3	D.5 page 131
56 - 75	166 to 180 cm	0 to 3	D.6 page 132

Table DD: 6 Weight Maintenance Tables for Women

Once you have selected the Weight Maintenance table that's appropriate for you, return to **Example 2** (page 44) for instruction on how to use the data in the table.

WEIGHT MAINTENANCE – WOMEN

Age: 18 to 35 yrs　　　　　　　　**Height: 150 to 165 cm**

Weight (kg)	ACTIVITY				
	Level 0	Level 1	Level 2	Level 3	Level 4
46	1740	1811	1971	2221	2700
48	1782	1857	2023	2284	2784
50	1824	1901	2074	2347	2867
52	1865	1945	2125	2408	2950
54	1905	1989	2176	2470	3032
56	1945	2032	2226	2531	3114
58	1985	2075	2275	2591	3195
60	2024	2117	2325	2651	3276
62	2063	2159	2373	2711	3356
64	2101	2200	2422	2770	3436
66	2139	2241	2470	2829	3516
68	2177	2282	2517	2888	3595
70	2214	2322	2565	2946	3674
75	2306	2422	2681	3090	3870
80	2396	2520	2797	3232	4065
85	2484	2616	2910	3373	4257
90	2571	2711	3022	3512	4449
95	2657	2804	3133	3650	4639
100	2741	2896	3242	3787	4827
105	2825	2987	3351	3922	5015
110	2907	3077	3458	4057	5202

Values in table are kcal per day.

Table D.1 Maintenance: Women 18 - 35, 150 - 165 cm

WEIGHT MAINTENANCE – WOMEN
Age: 18 to 35 yrs   Height: 166 - 180 cm

Weight (kg)	ACTIVITY				
	Level 0	Level 1	Level 2	Level 3	Level 4
46	1834	1905	2065	2315	2794
48	1878	1952	2118	2380	2879
50	1921	1999	2172	2444	2964
52	1964	2044	2224	2507	3049
54	2006	2090	2276	2570	3132
56	2047	2134	2328	2633	3216
58	2089	2178	2379	2695	3298
60	2129	2222	2430	2756	3381
62	2169	2265	2480	2818	3463
64	2209	2308	2530	2878	3544
66	2249	2351	2579	2938	3625
68	2288	2393	2628	2998	3706
70	2326	2435	2677	3058	3786
75	2421	2538	2797	3205	3986
80	2515	2639	2915	3351	4183
85	2606	2738	3032	3495	4379
90	2696	2836	3147	3637	4574
95	2785	2932	3261	3778	4767
100	2872	3027	3373	3917	4958
105	2958	3121	3484	4056	5148
110	3043	3213	3594	4193	5338
115	3127	3305	3703	4329	5526

Values in table are kcal per day.
Table D.2 Maintenance: Women 18 - 35, 166 - 180 cm

WEIGHT MAINTENANCE – WOMEN

Age: 36 to 55 yrs   **Height: 150 to 165 cm**

Weight (kg)	ACTIVITY			
	Level 0	Level 1	Level 2	Level 3
46	1693	1765	1924	2174
48	1735	1809	1975	2236
50	1775	1853	2026	2298
52	1815	1896	2076	2359
54	1855	1939	2126	2420
56	1894	1981	2175	2480
58	1933	2023	2224	2539
60	1971	2064	2272	2599
62	2009	2105	2320	2658
64	2047	2146	2368	2716
66	2084	2186	2415	2774
68	2121	2226	2462	2832
70	2158	2266	2508	2890
75	2248	2364	2624	3032
80	2336	2460	2737	3173
85	2423	2555	2849	3312
90	2509	2648	2960	3450
95	2593	2740	3069	3586
100	2676	2831	3177	3722
105	2758	2921	3284	3856
110	2839	3009	3390	3989

Values in table are kcal per day.

Table D.3   Maintenance: Women 36 - 55, 150 - 165 cm

WEIGHT MAINTENANCE – WOMEN

Age: 36 to 55 yrs   **Height: 166 to 180 cm**

Weight (kg)	ACTIVITY			
	Level 0	Level 1	Level 2	Level 3
46	1752	1823	1982	2233
48	1794	1869	2035	2296
50	1836	1913	2086	2359
52	1877	1958	2138	2421
54	1918	2002	2188	2482
56	1958	2045	2239	2544
58	1998	2088	2288	2604
60	2037	2130	2338	2664
62	2076	2172	2387	2724
64	2115	2214	2435	2784
66	2153	2255	2483	2843
68	2190	2296	2531	2901
70	2228	2336	2579	2960
75	2320	2436	2696	3104
80	2411	2535	2811	3247
85	2500	2631	2925	3388
90	2587	2726	3038	3528
95	2673	2820	3149	3666
100	2758	2913	3259	3803
105	2841	3004	3367	3939
110	2924	3094	3475	4074
115	3006	3184	3582	4208

Values in table are kcal per day.

Table D.4 Maintenance: Women 36 - 55, 166 - 180 cm

WEIGHT MAINTENANCE – WOMEN
Age: 56 to 75 yrs   Height: 150 to 165 cm

Weight (kg)	ACTIVITY			
	Level 0	Level 1	Level 2	Level 3
46	1619	1690	1849	2100
48	1659	1733	1899	2161
50	1698	1776	1949	2221
52	1737	1818	1998	2281
54	1775	1859	2046	2340
56	1813	1900	2094	2399
58	1851	1941	2142	2457
60	1888	1981	2189	2515
62	1925	2021	2236	2573
64	1961	2061	2282	2631
66	1998	2100	2328	2688
68	2033	2139	2374	2744
70	2069	2177	2420	2801
75	2156	2273	2532	2941
80	2242	2366	2643	3079
85	2327	2458	2753	3215
90	2410	2549	2861	3351
95	2492	2639	2968	3485
100	2573	2728	3074	3618
105	2652	2815	3178	3750
110	2731	2902	3282	3881

Values in table are kcal per day.

Table D.5 Maintenance: Women 56 - 75, 150 - 165 cm

WEIGHT MAINTENANCE – WOMEN

Age: 56 to 75 yrs   **Height: 166 to 180 cm**

Weight (kg)	ACTIVITY			
	Level 0	Level 1	Level 2	Level 3
46	1678	1749	1908	2159
48	1719	1793	1959	2220
50	1759	1836	2009	2282
52	1799	1879	2059	2343
54	1838	1922	2109	2403
56	1877	1964	2158	2463
58	1916	2006	2206	2522
60	1954	2047	2254	2581
62	1992	2088	2302	2640
64	2029	2128	2350	2698
66	2066	2168	2397	2756
68	2103	2208	2443	2814
70	2139	2247	2490	2871
75	2229	2345	2604	3013
80	2317	2441	2717	3153
85	2403	2535	2829	3292
90	2488	2627	2939	3429
95	2572	2719	3048	3565
100	2654	2809	3155	3700
105	2736	2898	3262	3834
110	2816	2987	3367	3966
115	2896	3074	3472	4098

Values in table are kcal per day.

Table D.6 Maintenance: Women 56 - 75, 166 - 180 cm

Appendix E Updated Weight Loss Model

At the time that Antonetti's weight-loss model was developed, the basil metabolic rate or the energy required to maintain the human body at rest was believed to best be represented by presuming it was dependent on body surface area [3]. But this assumption made the resulting weight loss predictive differential equation non-linear that required a relatively complex numerical solution using programmed software [4].

Then in 2016, professor Diana Thomas suggested the Antonetti model be updated by replacing the resting metabolic rate portion of the model with the much newer, validated and widely used Mifflin-St. Jeor regression equations [5]. As a bonus the update also eliminated the non-linearity in the Antonetti's original model and resulted in a differential equation with a much simpler closed-form solution, now called the Antonetti-Thomas weight loss model [6]. The most important advantage of the new Antonetti-Thomas model is that its solution is a relatively simple equation that can be used to directly solve practical weight loss prediction situations. (In fact, high-school algebra is all that is needed to use the Antonetti-Thomas model.) Before the new Antonetti-Thomas model is presented, however, some additional background is needed.

Physical Activity Energy (PA): This parameter has been shown to be directly proportional to an individual's weight. In other words for a given activity the more one weighs the more calories are burned. Expressed mathematically, $PA = KaW$, where Ka is the activity level coefficient and W is an individual's weight. Table 1 was adapted from [11]. The equivalent pedometer steps have been added by this writer.

Lifestyle	Ka (kcal/kg/d)	Approximate Daily Pedometer Steps
Sedentary	8	5000 or less
Light	10	About 6500
Moderate	13	About 8000
Vigorous	18	About 11500
Severe	27	17000 or more

Table 1: Activity Coefficient (*Ka*)

Resting Energy Expenditure: From Mifflin-St Jeor [5]:

For females: $B = 6.25H - 4.92A - 161$ For males: $B = 6.25H - 4.92A + 5$

where H is height (cm) and A is age (years). Two parameters that appear in the Antonetti-Thomas model are K_1 and K_2 which are defined as follows:

$K_1 = 0.9DI - B$ and $K_2 = Ka + 9.99$, where DI is dietary intake (kcal).

The derivation of the updated Antonetti-Thomas weight loss model is not covered here. (If interested in the details see Appendix F - Bibliography reference 6.) The Antonetti-Thomas model can be rearranged into three different versions to address the following types of problems:

1) Time to Lose Weight: How long will it take an individual to lose (or gain) a certain amount of weight. Solve for time:

$$ t = -\frac{\gamma}{K_2} \ln\left[\frac{K_1 - K_2 W_f}{K_1 - K_2 W_0} \right] \tag{1} $$

where t time on diet (days)
      γ energy value per unit of body mass lost = 7700 kcal/kg
      W_0 initial weight (kg)
      W_f final weight (kg)

2) Required Dietary Intake: What must the dietary intake of an individual be in order to lose (or gain) a certain amount of weight in a given amount of time? To solve for dietary intake use:

$$ DI = \frac{(-K_2 W_0 - B)\exp\left(-\dfrac{tK_2}{\gamma}\right) + K_2 W_f + B}{\left(\exp\left(-\dfrac{tK_2}{\gamma}\right) - 1\right)(-1+\alpha)} \tag{2} $$

where α specific dynamic action of food $= 0.10$

The Weight Loss Model is continued on the next page.

3) Amount of Weight Lost: And still another way of thinking about the problem is: How much weight will an individual lose (or gain) on a specified dietary intake in a given amount of time? To solve this type of problem use the following version of the Antonetti-Thomas model:

$$W_f = \frac{(K_2 W_0 - K_1)\exp\left(-\dfrac{tK_2}{\gamma}\right) + K_1}{K_2} \qquad (3)$$

$$\Delta W = W_0 - W_f \qquad (4)$$

PRACTICAL EXAMPLES

The following examples illustrate the use of the different versions of the Antonetti-Thomas model.

Example 1. How long will it take a <u>30 year-old female</u> on a 1200 kcal diet to lose 15 kg She weighs 85 kg, is 165 cm tall and is considered sedentary.

In this case we need to solve for the time (t) required to lose weight. Use equation 1.

where t time in days
       γ energy value per unit of mass, of body mass lost = 7700
       W_0 initial weight = 85 kg
       W_f final weight = 85 – 15 = 70 kg
       A age = 30 years
       Ka activity level = 8 kcal/kg/day (from Table 1 for sedentary)
       H height = 165 cm

For 30-year old female:

$$B = 6.25H - 4.92A - 161 = 6.25(165) - 4.92(30) - 161 = 722.7$$

$$K_1 = 0.9DI - B = 0.9(1200) - 722.7 = 1080 - 722.7 = 357.3 \;,$$

$$K_2 = Ka + 9.99 = 8.0 + 9.99 = 17.99$$

Substitute above values for all parameters into equation 1:

$$t = -\frac{\gamma}{K_2} ln\left[\frac{K_1 - K_2 W_f}{K_1 - K_2 W_0}\right] = -\frac{7700}{17.99} ln\left[\frac{357.3 - 17.99(70)}{357.3 - 17.99(85)}\right] = 112 \text{ days}$$

<u>Example 2.</u> Determine the dietary intake required for a 30-year old female to lose 15 kg in 100 days. She is 165 cm tall, weighs 90 kg and her activity level is thought to be light. From Table 1, $Ka = 10.0$. (<u>This example is particularly useful for nutritionists and dieticians.</u>)

In this case we need to solve for the dietary intake (DI) required to lose a given amount of weight and we use equation 2.

$K_2 = 10.0 + 9.99 = 19.99$, As in example 1, $B = 722.7$, $\gamma = 7700$, $\alpha = 0.10$ but $W_0 = 90$ kg, $W_f = 75$ kg and $t = 100$ days. Substitute these values into equation 2.

$$DI = \frac{(-19.99(90) - 722.7)\exp\left\{-\frac{100(19.99)}{7700}\right\} + 19.99(75) + 722.7}{(\exp\left\{-\frac{100(19.99)}{7700}\right\} - 1)(-1 + 0.10)} = 1345 \text{ kcal/d}$$

Thus this dieter should eat 1345 kcal per day to lose 15 kg in 100 days.

<u>Example 3.</u> How much weight will a 60-year old male on 1200 kcal diet lose in 100 days? He weighs 95 kg, is 178 cm tall and is considered moderately active.

For 60-year old male:

$$B = 6.25H - 4.92A + 5 = 6.25(165) - 4.92(60) + 5 = 741.1$$

$$K_1 = 0.9DI - B = 0.9(1200) - 741.1 = 1080 - 741.1 = 338.9$$

$Ka = 13.0$ (from Table 1 for moderately active)

$$K_2 = Ka + 9.99 = 13.0 + 9.99 = 22.99$$

In this case we need to solve for his final weight (W_f) after 100 days on a 1200 kcal diet. Use equation 3. Substitute the appropriate values into equation 3:

$$W_f = \frac{(22.99(95) - 338.9)\exp\left(-\frac{100(22.99)}{7700}\right) + 338.9}{22.99} = 74.3 \text{ kg}$$

Then the amount of weight this man would lose is given by equation 4:

$$\Delta W = W_0 - W_f = 95 - 74.3 = 20.7 \text{ kg}$$

Summary   The new Antonetti-Thomas weight loss predictive model provides a simple, straight-forward method to calculate realistic weight loss for an individual or at a population-wide level.

Appendix F Bibliography

1.   Atwater and F.G. Benedict 1903 Experiments on the metabolism of matter and energy in the human body. U.S. Dept Agriculture Exptl. Sta. Bull. 136.
2. Antonetti, V.W. 1973 The equations governing weight change in human beings. *Am J Clin Nutr* 26 (1):64-71.
3. Bruen, C. 1930 Variation of basal metabolic rate per unit surface area with age. *J Gen Physiol* 13 (6):607-610.
4. Antonetti, V.W. 1973 *The Computer Diet: A Weight Control Guide*. New York, M. Evans.
5. Mifflin, M.D., S.T. St. Jeor, et al. 1990 A new predictive equation for resting energy expenditure in healthy individuals. *J Clin Nutr* 51 (2):241-247.
6. Thomas, D.M. and V.W. Antonetti. Dynamic modeling of energy expenditure to estimate Dietary Energy Intake. from Schoeller, D.A. and M. Westerterp-Plantenga,ed. 2017 *Advances in the Assessment of Dietary Intake.* New York, CRC Press, Chapter 12: 211-219.
7. Westerterp, K.R., et al. 1995 Energy intake, physical activity and body weight: A simulation model. *Br J Nutr* 73 (3):337-347.
8. Hall, K.D. 2010 Predicting metabolic adaptation, body weight change, and energy intake in humans. *Am J Endrocrinol Metab* 298(3):E449-E466.
9. Thomas, D.M., et al. 2011 A simple model predicting weight change in humans. *J Bio Dyn* 5 (6):579-599.
10. Thomas, D.M., et al. 2014 Time to correctly predict the amount of weight loss with dieting. *J Acad Nutr Diet* 114 (6):857.
11. Taylor, C.M. and O.F. Pye. *Foundations of Nutrition*. New York, Macmillan, 1966, p. 48.
12. Moran, M.J., et al. *Fundamentals of Engineering Thermodynamics*, New York, Wiley, 2014.

Disclaimer

This book offers general weight control information. It is not a medical manual and the author does not claim to be medically qualified. The material in this book is not intended to be a substitute for medical counseling. Everyone should have a medical checkup before beginning a weight loss program. Moreover, the physician conducting the medical exam should be made aware of and should approve the specific weight control program planned. Additionally, while the author and publisher have made every effort to ensure the accuracy of the information in this book, they make no representations or warranties regarding its accuracy or completeness. Further, neither the author nor publisher assume liability for any medical problems that might result from applying the methods in this book, or for any loss of profit, or any other commercial damages, including but not limited to special, incidental, consequential or other damages, and any such liability is hereby expressly disclaimed.

<u>NoPaperPress eBooks and Paperbacks</u>

100-Day Super Diet-1200 Cal*
100-Day Super Diet-1500 Cal*
100-Day No-Cooking Diet-1200 Cal*
100-Day No-Cooking Diet-1500 Cal*
90-Day Smart Diet-1200 Cal*
90-Day Smart Diet-1500 Cal*
90-Day No-Cooking Diet - 1200 Cal*
90-Day No-Cooking Diet - 1500 Cal*
90-Day Perfect Diet - 1200 Cal*
90-Day Perfect Diet - 1500 Cal*
60-Day Perfect Diet-1200 Cal*
60-Day Perfect Diet-1500 Cal*
50-Day Flex Diet-1200 Cal*
50-Day Flex Diet-1500 Cal*
30-Day Quick Diet - Women*
30-Day Quick Diet for Men*
30-Day No-Cooking Diet*
30-Day Diet - Women - Metric*
30-Day Diet for Men - Metric*
25 Day Easy Diet-1200 Cal*
25 Day Easy Diet-1500 Cal*
25-Day No-Cooking Diet
10-Day Express Diet
10-Day No-Cooking Diet*
7-Day Diet for Women*
7-Day Diet for Men*
7-Day No-Cooking Diets*
90-Day Gluten-Free Diet-1200 Cal*
90-Day Gluten-Free Diet-1500 Cal*
30-Day Gluten-Free Quick Diet*
30-Day Gluten-Free No-Cooking Diet*
7-Day Diet for Women - Metric*
7-Day Diet for Men - Metric
7-Day Gluten-Free Express Diet*
7-Day Gluten-Free No-Cooking Diet*
90-Day Vegetarian Diet-1200 Cal*
90-Day Vegetarian Diet-1500 Cal*
30-Day Vegetarian Diet*
7-Day Vegetarian Diet*
Weight Loss for Women*
Weight Loss for Women - Metric
Weight Loss for Women - UK
Weight Loss for Men*
Maximum Weight Loss - 1200 Cal*
Maximum Weight Loss - 1500 Cal*

Weight Loss for Men - Metric*
Maximum Weight Loss- 1200 Cal*
Maximum Weight Loss- 1500 Cal*
Weight Control - U.S. Edition*
Weight Control - Metric. Edition
Prof Weight Control Women - U.S.
Prof Weight Control Women - Metric
Prof Weight Control Men - U.S.
Prof Weight Control Men - Metric
Weight Maintenance - U.S. Ed*
Weight Maintenance - Metric. Ed*
Weight Maintenance - UK Ed
Weight Loss for Senior Men*
Weight Loss for Senior Women*
Eat Smart - U.S. Edition*
Eat Smart - Metric Edition
30-Day Mediterranean Diet
Exercise Smart - U.S. Edition*
Exercise Smart - Metric Edition
Exercise Smart - UK Edition*
Total Fitness - U.S. Edition
Total Fitness - Metric Edition
Total Fitness - UK Edition
Total Fitness for Women-U.S. Ed*
Total Fitness for Women - Metric
Total Fitness for Women - UK Ed
Total Fitness for Men - U.S. Ed*
Total Fitness for Men- Metric Ed*
Total Fitness for Men - UK Ed
Senior Fitness - U.S. Edition*
Senior Fitness - Metric Edition*
Senior Fitness - UK Edition*
Computer Diet - U.S. Edition*
Computer Diet - Metric Ed*
Reliable Weight Loss - U.S. Ed
101 Weight Loss Tips*
101 Healthy Eating Tips*
101 Lifelong Fitness Tips*
101 Weight Maintenance Tips
101 Weight Loss Recipes
101 GF Weight Loss Recipes
101 Veggie Weight Loss Recipes*
30-Day Mediterranean Diet*
90-Day Mediterranean Diet - 1200 Cal*
90-Day Mediterranean Diet - 1500 Cal*

* These titles are available as both ebooks and paperbacks. Our ebooks are sold by Amazon, Apple, Google, Barnes & Noble and Kobo, but our paperbacks are only sold by Amazon.

www.ingramcontent.com/pod-product-compliance
Lightning Source LLC
Chambersburg PA
CBHW051459250726
48655CB00001B/488